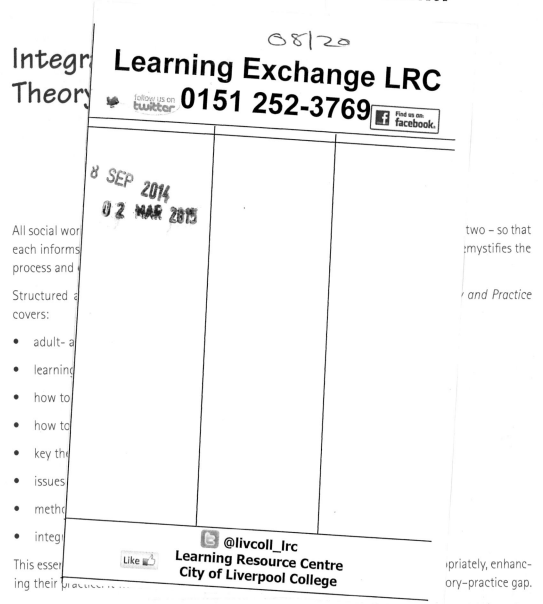

Integr...
Theory...

All social wor... two – so that
each informs... mystifies the
process and ...

Structured a... and Practice
covers:

- adult- a...
- learning...
- how to...
- how to...
- key the...
- issues...
- metho...
- integr...

This esser... priately, enhanc-
ing their practice... ory-practice gap.

Pam Green Lister is Director of the Masters in Social Work at the Glasgow School of Social Work. She teaches social work theory and practice and has researched widely within social work education.

Student Social Work

This exciting new textbook series is ideal for all students studying to be qualified social workers, whether at undergraduate or masters level. Covering key elements of the social work curriculum, the books are accessible, interactive and thought-provoking.

New titles

Human Growth and Development
John Sudbery

Mental Health Social Work in Context
Nick Gould

Social Work and Social Policy
An introduction
Jonathan Dickens

Social Work Placements
Mark Doel

Social Work
A reader
Viviene E. Cree

Sociology for Social Workers and Probation Officers
Viviene E. Cree

Integrating Social Work Theory and Practice
A practical skills guide
Pam Green Lister

Forthcoming titles

Social Work Law and Ethics
Jonathan Dickens

Social Work with Children and Young People, their Families and Carers
Janet Warren

Becoming a Social Worker, 2nd edn
Narratives from around the world
Viviene E. Cree

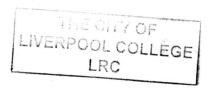
Integrating Social Work Theory and Practice

A practical skills guide

Pam Green Lister

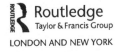 Routledge
Taylor & Francis Group

LONDON AND NEW YORK

First published 2012
by Routledge
2 Park Square, Milton Park, Abingdon, Oxon, OX14 4RN

Simultaneously published in the USA and Canada
by Routledge
711 Third Avenue, New York, NY 10017

Routledge is an imprint of the Taylor & Francis Group, an informa business

British Library Cataloguing in Publication Data
A catalogue record for this book is available from the British Library

Library of Congress Cataloging-in-Publication Data
Lister, Pam Green.
  Integrating social work theory and practice : a practical skills guide/ Pam Green Lister. — 1st ed.
    p. cm.
  1. Social service. I. Title.
  HV11.L54 2012
  361.301—dc23   2011029422

ISBN13: 978-0-415-48112-0 (hbk)
ISBN13: 978-0-415-48113-7 (pbk)
ISBN13: 978-0-203-13651-5 (ebk)

Designed and typeset in Rotis
by Keystroke, Station Road, Codsall, Wolverhampton

Printed and bound in Great Britain by the MPG Books Group

Contents

Contents

Contents

Acknowledgements

I would like to thank colleagues and students at the Glasgow School of Social Work, with whom I have worked on research in social work education. This collaborative work has formed the basis for this book.

1 Introduction

Social work education requires students to demonstrate the ability to integrate theory and practice in academic and practice learning settings in a critically reflective and anti-oppressive way. This text aims to offer some guidance on how you might develop these skills. The focus of the book is on the 'how to', so you will be introduced to a range of techniques and frameworks, which have been developed as a result of undertaking research into social work education with colleagues and students. The book is aimed at students at the start of their social work education. It is not a compendium of theories in social work but concentrates on the development of study skills. Therefore, in each chapter some social work texts are focused on in more detail to demonstrate how the material in the texts may be used. At the end of each chapter you are encouraged to complete exercises to assist you to develop these skills.

Chapter 2 introduces students to the concepts of adult- and student-centred learning. It will examine learning styles before giving an overview of what might be expected on a social work programme. A range of learning and teaching methods will be discussed, followed by an outline of the main methods of assessment that you might encounter on your course.

In Chapter 3 reflection, criticality and transfer of learning are examined, with reference to research undertaken with students in this area. A series of vignettes will be provided to show how the core concepts can be applied in practice.

How and where to look for theoretical explanations is discussed in the fourth chapter. It is acknowledged that, when asked to apply theory to practice, students often find it difficult to navigate through the large amount of social work and social work-related texts. You will be introduced to the key principles of inquiry drawn from research literature, and then to the process of problem-based learning. A framework for analysing social work texts will be suggested.

Anti-oppressive theory and practice is an area which often causes concern in students. Sometimes they are uncertain as to how they can demonstrate this, and it is viewed primarily as purely taking action. It is important that you understand the underlying concepts and the process of anti-oppressive practice. Therefore, there are two chapters which address the issues of anti-oppressive theory and practice. Chapter 5 presents core concepts such as social division, power and anti-oppressive ethics. Chapter 6 examines the processes of anti-oppressive practice such as empowerment, advocacy and service user and carer involvement.

Chapter 7 offers ways in which you might approach the integration of theory and practice in social work assessments. A range of definitions and purposes are presented, followed by an overview of the processes involved in assessment. You are presented with the outcomes of research into the ways in which textbooks address assessment in the form of two frameworks, to assist in the critical analysis of those texts.

Methods of intervention are introduced in Chapter 8 where you are introduced to two of them – psychosocial social work and task-centred work – by showing how the study of three key social work texts can provide a solid foundation from which to understand these methods. You are guided through how you might gain an initial understanding of methods by reading and analysing core texts. You are then encouraged to further your understanding using the framework outlined in Chapter 4.

Chapters 9 and 10 draw significantly from research with students. It is hoped that by demonstrating to you how other students were involved in research you may be encouraged to develop your own methods which will assist in the critical integration of theory and practice. Chapter 9 critiques a third method of intervention, solution-focused social work, using a Critical Analysis Framework tool initially developed and evaluated by social work students. Solution-focused social work was chosen as the method to be critiqued as students can find its core concepts and methods difficult to understand. The chapter provides an example of how this framework might be used in practice.

Chapter 10 introduces you to a further tool, Critical Incident Analysis, also developed with students and practice teachers/assessors, to assist the development of criticality. Students' evaluations of the Critical Incident Framework are given and an extended example from one student is provided.

The processes, frameworks and tools presented in this book are ways in which students, at the beginning of their social work education, might begin to integrate theory and practice. There is concern in social work about the proliferation of tools and guidance which inhibit creativity and professional development in all aspects of the profession. My intention in this book is not to add to this proliferation of rigid tools. Rather it is to provide suggestions as to how you might begin to integrate theory and practice from the very beginning of your social work education.

2 Learning processes

In this chapter you will be introduced to some core educational concepts and processes. Basic components of a social work degree will be explained, and an overview of learning, teaching and assessment methods used in social work education will be given.

Adult- and student-centred learning

Knowles (1978) is credited with developing the concept of 'adult learning', and with the application of this concept to social work education. He criticised the dominant model of 'pedagogy' which, he suggested, framed the learning process in terms of an expert teacher transmitting knowledge to a novice learner. This way of understanding the learning and teaching process is often described as being based on the premise that learners are empty vessels which need to be filled. Knowles argued that for adults to learn effectively, and to the best of their ability, they must be involved in identifying their own learning needs, planning the process of learning and designing learning experiences. The role of the teacher is to provide learning opportunities, which involve experiential techniques and attention to practice applications appropriate to the stage of student learning, to facilitate this process in a safe learning environment.

Building on the work of Knowles (1978) and others, Entwistle (1987, 1990) identified the ingredients of 'student-centred learning'. He made explicit what might seem an obvious process, that students require adequate prior knowledge and understanding before learning can take place, and that the content of the learning and teaching should match the intellectual stage of the student. The role of the teacher is to assist students to see the relevance of learning and encourage them to take a reflexive approach to study. Teaching strategies would include modelling, creating opportunities for discussion and providing feedback. The aim of this approach is to facilitate 'deep' as opposed to 'surface' learning. 'Surface' learning is typified by rote learning and an uncritical acquisition of knowledge which is used strategically, for example to fulfil an assessment task, and then not revisited. A student adopting a 'deep' approach to learning would develop a more in-depth understanding of concepts, seeking to comprehend the theoretical principles behind concepts and then make connections between newly acquired and previous knowledge and experience.

Walker (2008) characterises an autonomous learner as having an 'engaged disposition towards learning' (Walker 2008: 98). An active learner is active, not merely receptive, a person who does not merely reproduce information but identifies relationships, identifies their own learning goals, uses feedback but is also self-monitoring and develops their own learning resources and strategies.

Learning styles

There has been extensive research into the different styles adopted by learners. A range of learning styles inventories has been produced to assist students to identify their particular learning style (Kolb 1976; Dunn 1996). With this awareness students can then devise study strategies which suit their learning needs. The most well known Learning Styles Questionnaire used in social work education in the UK was devised by Honey and Mumford (1992). The questionnaire consists of a series of statements with which students are asked to agree or disagree. Some examples of the statements are:

- What matters most is whether something works in practice.

- I take care over the interpretation of data available to me and avoid jumping to conclusions.

- I like to ponder many alternatives before making up my mind.

These statements are chosen to help students tease out their approach to learning. The authors stress that there is no right or wrong answer, just as there are no right or wrong ways of learning. On completion of the questionnaire students then score their responses in a table. The statements are organised into four columns, entitled Activist, Reflector, Theorist and Pragmatist. By simply ticking which statements they agreed with students produce a score in each column which indicates what type of learner they are. Honey and Mumford (1992) provide a general description of the four learning styles and suggest learning activities which best suit a learning style. These are summarised in Table 2.1.

Completing the Learning Styles Questionnaire and identifying the learning style/s which most accurately describes your approach to learning can be a useful first step in building study skills. Clearly, the above four categories are very general ones which can provide pointers on how to structure your

Table 2.1
Learning styles

Learning style	Learn best where:	Learn least from:
Activists: • involve themselves fully; • operate in the 'here and now'; • challenged by new experiences but may bore easily.	• there are new experiences; • they are thrown in at the deep end; • there are diverse activities.	• a learning activity which is passive and/or repetitive; • engaging in solitary work; • being asked to analyse and synthesise lots of data.
Reflectors: • examine experiences from a number of perspectives; • thoroughly analyse data before reaching a conclusion; • cautious.	• time is allowed to think over activities; • they can carry out research; • they are asked to produce careful analysis.	• being forced into the limelight; • they have no time to plan; • they are given insufficient data and time.
Theorists: • integrate observations into logical theories; • like to analyse and synthesise; • detached and analytical.	• they have time to explore a problem methodically; • they are intellectually stretched; • they can analyse and generalise.	• being involved in unstructured activities; • being set a problem without a context or apparent purpose; • where they find the subject matter lacks depth.
Pragmatists: • keen to try out new ideas; • experimental; • like to get on with things.	• there is a clear link between the subject matter and a task; • they are shown techniques with practical advantages; • they are given opportunities to practise.	• the learning is not related to an immediate need; • there is no practice or clear guidelines; • they cannot see sufficient reward for the learning activity.

learning activities. However, it is likely that most students can identify elements of all four learning styles, and the particular approach to learning is dependent on the context. Honey and Mumford's (1992) Learning Styles Questionnaire has been criticised in that it was devised through working with managers and no information is given with regard to the gender and ethnicity of the groups. Caution is also desirable because their identification of discrete learning styles tends to suggest that a learning style is fixed and static, and that different approaches to learning cannot be developed (Doel and Shardlow 2005). As we will see below, there are a range of methods of learning, teaching and assessment used in social work education which may facilitate your learning, across the learning style spectrum.

The core components of a social work degree

In order for social work courses to be validated by the regulatory body, the courses have to demonstrate that they have met the statutory requirements of that body across the course as a whole. Courses must also be validated by the universities and have to demonstrate that the courses are constructed around the benchmark statements which specify the assessment levels which must be met at each stage of the undergraduate degree. Social work courses comprise both learning and teaching, which take place both in the university and in practice learning. Courses are usually composed of individual modules, the learning and teaching content and the assessment of which are planned across the course of the degree.

Practice learning

Practice learning is, of course, a core component of social work education. A period of assessed practice learning is often referred to as a placement. In the UK you are assessed prior to your first practice learning opportunity in order to ensure that you are ready to practice. In the period of practice learning, you have to demonstrate core skills and meet required standards and learning outcomes in working with service users, carers and other professionals. You will be supervised by a practice teacher or assessor, who will report on your practice. Students produce evidence of their learning in an assessed assignment. This assessment tool may take a variety of forms.

Individual modules

In constructing individual modules social work educators take cognisance of the level at which the module will be assessed. They decide on the overall aims of the module, learning outcomes (i.e. what students are expected to have learned by the end of the module), module content and how this meets requirements, methods of delivery of course content and method/s of assessment. Indicative reading is given to support private study. The aim of designing a module is that there is a relationship between what is taught in the module, how it is taught, and the method of assessment.

Methods of learning and teaching

In your social work course you will experience diverse learning and teaching methods. Depending on your own approach to learning you may find that some methods are more interesting or challenging than others. The following section summarises the most common learning and teaching methods used in a classroom setting and indicates the differing purposes of the methods.

Lectures/didactic teaching

The word 'didactic' stems from the Greek word for 'teach' and is also defined as 'intended to instruct' and 'having instruction as an ulterior purpose' (OED). In most courses or modules a series of lectures will form the backbone of the learning experience. Typically lectures aim to give an overview of the subject. The aim would be to highlight key themes and issues to provide a starting point for further study. Lecturers will summarise relevant research and guide students towards further reading. A common concern among students is that lectures do not cover all aspects of a topic. The purpose of a lecture is not to provide a definitive account of a subject but rather to provide a stimulus for more in-depth study.

Seminars

A seminar is 'a small class at a university etc. for discussion and research' and a 'class meeting for systematic study under the direction of a specified person' (OED). Seminars are guided group discussions in which topics can be examined in more depth. Usually, the topic relates to a previous lecture and affords students the opportunity to check their understanding, offer explanations and exchange ideas. You are expected to prepare to contribute to the seminar by undertaking tasks such as guided reading. Participation in the seminar itself might consist of contributing to a discussion or making a short presentation. The lecturer is responsible for the process of the seminar, ensuring that key areas are discussed and that all students are able to contribute. The lecturer may instigate discussion by putting forward a proposition or asking direct questions of students.

Small group work

There are several forms of small group work. It may take place within a longer lecture, for example a lecturer may outline key themes and then ask students to discuss them in small informal groups. It may also be timetabled in a more structured way, for example you may meet on a weekly basis to discuss and research a specific area. Such group work may be project-based and lead to assessed or non-assessed presentations. Small group work offers students the opportunity to create their own learning programme. By working in small groups you can develop communication skills and build confidence in making presentations. In order to provide a fruitful opportunity for learning, it is important that you develop the skills of listening, presenting ideas succinctly and giving feedback. Small groups offer the opportunity to share and clarify ideas and learn from others' experience and knowledge. There is sometimes a misconception among students that learning only takes place when a lecturer is present when, for learning to take place, it is the learner who has to be present.

Skills groups

The development of good communication skills is a key learning aim of social work courses. These skills include those of listening, using appropriate verbal and non-verbal communication, preparing for contact with a service user or professional, interviewing, gathering and analysing information, planning work with the service user, and ending contact. In order to assist students to develop and rehearse good communication skills social work educators engage students in skills rehearsal. Skills rehearsal includes a variety of individual and group activities which usually involve various kinds of role play.

Problem-based learning

Problem-based learning (PBL) is a method of learning and teaching which relies on both independent study and research, and small group work. It is also called Enquiry and Action Learning. There are various models of PBL. Some entire courses/modules are based on the method, whereas in other courses/modules PBL forms one part of study. Typically, PBL groups are staffed, although the staff member does not take responsibility for the process and content of the discussion, but intervenes only if the discussion is veering seriously off course or if clarification of an issue is required. The group chooses a chair and a scribe for each group session. A PBL group usually begins with students being given a case scenario and a trigger statement. Students discuss the scenario and statement and identify 'problems' or areas that require further research. Tasks are then allocated and students research their chosen area, and present findings the following week, after which another trigger statement is given to the group to stimulate further study. PBL group work has the same advantages as more informal group work discussed above. In addition it affords you the opportunity to develop the skills of chairing, scribing and reporting back. The process of PBL assists you to develop critical thinking and research skills.

Tutorials

Traditionally social work courses have developed tutorial systems which involve substantially more one-to-one contact with students compared to many other courses in the field of social science, for example. Tutors meet regularly with students on an individual or group basis and have an overview of your progress both within the university and in practice learning. Tutorials offer you the opportunity to discuss your learning needs and achievements and may include discussion of individual assignments or specific issues which arise in practice learning. The focus of tutorials is on academic support but students are usually encouraged to alert tutors to any wider issue which may be affecting their learning.

Individual/private study

A student is defined as a 'person engaged in or fond of study'. The verb 'to study' derives from the Latin for 'to be zealous and apply oneself' (OED). It is further defined as 'to apply the mind to acquiring knowledge, especially devoting time and effort to this end' (OED). Time and effort are the core components of individual study. In all social work courses/modules, student contact time is calculated (that is, time in classes, be it lectures, seminars or groups with a lecturer). However, your effort (i.e. the number of hours you should study individually) is also calculated and it is usually expected that the majority of hours in any module is used in private study. Private study encompasses a range of activity including organising academic work, searching the literature in the library and online, reading, note taking, writing assignments, preparing presentations and revising for exams. Private study is central to work within the university and work when in practice learning.

Online study

Online study is becoming increasingly important in social work education. Alongside administrative information about the course and individual modules, you may be required to study online by engaging in such activities as group discussion, posting your research to fellow students, completing question-naires, quizzes, examinations, and working through interactive scenarios. Some modules may consist mainly of online study while others may use it in conjunction with other methods, for example problem-based learning, discussed above.

Assessment

Assessment in social work education has a variety of purposes. Its ultimate purpose is to determine if a student is fit to enter the profession of social work. It measures the extent to which students have achieved the learning outcomes of the course or module. Throughout the course you have to undertake a range of assessment tasks to demonstrate this achievement. Feedback is given on the work produced for assessment, and this can assist you in identifying future learning needs.

There are a range of methods used to assess students in social work education (Crisp and Green Lister 2002; Green Lister, Dutton and Crisp 2005). The most frequently used assessment methods found in the research of the above authors are outlined below.

Essays

Most students will be familiar with writing essays. The term 'essay' is derived from the Latin term to denote an 'attempt or endeavour', and developed to mean 'a short prose composition on any subject' and 'a first attempt at learning, composition' (OED). This suggests that a prime aim of the essay is to give students the opportunity to demonstrate how they are beginning to understand a subject by means of a short written script. You can demonstrate your individual understanding of a topic and your writing skills. Essays require you to research the topic provided by the essay question and then demonstrate your understanding of the subject by analysing the material and developing a coherent argument. In doing so you must be clear about the requirements of the essay question, collect and record information, plan how you will address the essay question and then present the analysed material in an integrated way.

Examinations

Examinations may be in a written, oral, or computerised form. Written examinations may take the form of several short essays or a multiple choice paper. Most examinations take place within the university and students are asked to complete the assessment task in a finite time. The examination papers are often 'unseen', i.e. students have not seen the questions. They may also be 'seen' in that students are given the assignment task, have time to research the topic and must then answer the questions in a finite time in the university. Examinations also differ in how much material can be used as a resource within the exam. Written examinations serve the purpose of allowing you to show that you can recall knowledge, demonstrate understanding, think critically and write effectively under time-restricted conditions. Oral examinations serve a similar purpose to written examinations, but may also be a form of assessment of presentational skills. Computerised examinations are most frequently used to test Information Technology (IT) skills in social work education. As students develop IT skills, further use may be made of this method of assessment.

Presentations

Presentations may be made individually, as a group, or by poster. In social work practice it is important to be able to present an argument in various forums. Assessed presentations differ from oral examinations in that students choose or are given a topic to research with time to prepare. Oral presentations are usually assessed for content and for presentation skills such as coherency, visual aids and ability to respond to questions. Poster presentations demonstrate visual presentational skills but might also involve an assessment of an explanation of the content of the poster.

Learning logs, journals and reflective diaries

The terms journals, learning logs and reflective diaries are used to describe an ongoing written account of learning. A structure may be prescribed, in that you are given a pro forma structure to follow, or you may be allowed to determine your own structure. As a learning tool, learning logs assist you to record your learning. The emphasis is not only on recording what you did but why and how you did it, the aim of which is to assist you to reflect on and critically analyse what you are doing. Learning logs can be used in course work and are a common tool in the assessment of practice learning. They may be requested as part of a portfolio.

Critical Incident Analysis

Critical Incident Analysis is similar to a learning log in that the aim is to assist students to describe, reflect and analyse. However, as the name suggests, in Critical Incident Analysis you would focus on a specific critical incident from which you think you have learned. Usually Critical Incident Analysis is structured and you are prompted to reflect on particular questions. Like learning logs, Critical Incident Analysis can be used both in the university and in practice learning, and may be required as part of a portfolio. Critical Incident Analysis is discussed in detail in Chapter 10.

Course work assignments

The term course work assignment is used to describe a series of assessments which take place throughout a module. In this method of assessment, rather than students completing one assessment at the end of the module, they are required to submit a number of smaller pieces of work. These pieces of work might include other methods discussed here such as essays (in a shortened version), a learning log, a critical incident analysis or a small computerised examination. These assessments may be presented at the end of the module in the form of portfolios, which are discussed below.

Videoed role plays

As well as being a frequently used learning and teaching method, role plays, especially those that are video recorded, are used as an assessment instrument. The role plays are usually based around a simulated interview with a service user. Increasingly service users and carers act as the interviewee. They may be assessed by a member of the university staff, a social work professional, a service user or a carer. A reflective commentary is often provided by the student. In this commentary the student is asked to reflect upon and analyse their skills, identifying areas in which they show strength and those which need to be developed. This form of assessment is used in a number of courses as the means by which you demonstrate that you are ready to undertake your first period of practice learning.

Reports

Reports of work undertaken are used in both university and practice learning settings. Reports are a record of work or research. A report of research would typically give an overview of the literature in the subject and of previous research in the area to be researched. It would describe and analyse the methods used to gather information for the topic of study. An analysis of the data gathered would then be presented and conclusions and recommendations would follow. This process is similar to that involved in undertaking dissertations. Reports produced as evidence of the learning outcomes of practice learning are based on an account of work undertaken on placement. You would be expected to describe, reflect on and analyse learning with reference to key roles and standards.

Portfolios

Portfolios are widely used in social work education. They can be used to demonstrate learning in a particular module, in a period of practice learning or an entire course. Portfolios comprise a number of elements and all of the above forms of assessment may appear in a portfolio. The content may be more or less prescribed. Portfolios give you the opportunity to demonstrate your learning in a variety of formats and present very different elements of your work.

Dissertations

Dissertations are 'a spoken or written subject in which it is treated at length' (OED). In social work education, dissertations may be based on an empirical piece of research which is based on observation and experiment, or a literature-based experiment which is based on analysis of the theory and literature in the field of study. They are usually undertaken towards the end of a course and you choose your own topic of study. Students undertake a period of supervised study leading to the production of a dissertation. Individual universities have developed specific regulations and guidance for dissertations.

Exercise 1

Consider the summary of Honey and Mumford's Learning Styles Questionnaire (1992) described above.

- From the outline given, which learning style or styles do you think best describes how you learn?

- What reason can you give for this? Note down some examples from your previous studies.

Exercise 2

A range of learning, teaching and assessment methods has been presented in this chapter. Having begun to consider your learning style, consider:

- Which learning and teaching methods do you think best suit your learning needs and why?

- Which learning and teaching methods do you think least suit your learning needs and why?

- Which assessment methods do you think best suit your learning needs and why?

- Which assessment methods do you think least suit your learning needs and why?

- What plans do you need to make in order to make use of the learning and teaching and assessment methods which least suit your learning needs?

Key learning points

- Social work education is based on the student being an active learner.

- Having an awareness of your learning style/s can help you to consider how you might approach academic or practice situations.

- There are a range of learning and teaching and assessment methods, each with their own benefits and challenges. Knowing this can assist you in engaging with a particular learning and teaching or assessment activity.

Further reading

Crisp, B.R. and Green Lister, P. (2002) 'Assessment methods in social work education: A review of the literature', *Social Work Education*, 21(2): 259–69.

Doel, M. and Shardlow, S.M. (2005) *Modern social work practice*, Aldershot: Ashgate.

3 Reflection, criticality and transfer of learning

While in the discussion of learning styles previously it was acknowledged that students enter education with different learning styles, a key aim of social work education is to encourage you to become a *reflective* and *critical* practitioner and to be able to *transfer* previous learning and experience to new learning situations. In doing so, you will demonstrate an ability to integrate theory and practice. This chapter will define these terms and discuss how these skills can be developed throughout the social work course.

Reflection

Reflection can be defined as 'the action of turning (back) or fixing one's thoughts on some subject' and 'the process or faculty by which the mind has knowledge of itself and its own workings' (OED). Reflection in learning is a cyclical and continuous process which involves experiencing an event, returning to that experience, reflecting upon it, and in doing so attending to feelings, identifying learning and then re-evaluating the experience. It is suggested that for successful learning to take place learners must *reflect in and on action* (Schön 1983). Reflection may consist of reflective thinking which is not directly expressed but informs future thinking and action; reflective discussion, for example with a practice supervisor; or reflective writing for academic or practice purposes.

Walker (2008: 87) summarises the important ingredients of reflection as:

- intellectual activity – thinking;

- affective activity – feeling or experiencing emotions;

- using these to explore or find out more about experiences;

- the result of which should be different and fresh thinking.

She suggests that reflection requires the deep approach to learning described by Entwistle (1987). In reflection workers have to articulate their experience and how they 'went about things' (Walker 2008: 87). A reflective practitioner welcomes doubt, uncertainty and contradictions. As a result, a reflective practitioner is an active participant in the use and development of their own knowledge. Professional decision making is aided by being exposed to thinking from a different angle and is aided by developing understanding and self-awareness of your own thinking, and this new understanding will improve professional practice.

Walker also argues that reflection in social work is important as it assists the processes of thinking through and articulating decisions, and this means that the social worker can be held accountable for such decisions, which may be based on particular values and assumptions. The risk of routine responses is avoided and reflection aids workers to move beyond their current ways of thinking. It also assists workers to consider the impact of self on the situation.

Criticality

There are numerous aspects of criticality. The concept encompasses critical thinking, critical questioning, critical reading, critical writing, critical reasoning, and critical practice. As will be shown below, these aspects of criticality are not mutually exclusive but rather emphasise the different processes of the concept of criticality.

Critical thinking has been defined as the 'skilled, active, interpretation and evaluation of observations, communications, information and argumentation, as a guide to thought and action' (Fisher and Scriven 1997: 20).

Walker (2008: 59–60) provides a useful summary of research on critical thinking which suggests that in order to develop critical thinking a person must:

- take a questioning and sceptical stance;

- aim for a deep understanding of knowledge and complex ideas; this includes an appreciation of the context of the ideas, their history, their construction, and their relationships to other knowledge and means not seeing knowledge as a series of facts;

- explore a range of alternative ideas;

- identify and challenge the assumptions that underlie ideas;

- examine the evidence for knowledge and ideas;

- recognise the role of feelings when working with ideas;

- be able to use ideas to make an argument and an informed judgement;

- take a critical stance towards their own process of thinking.

Jones (2009) offers a typology of aspects to criticality: developing critical questions; developing critical reading; developing critical writing; developing critical reasoning; and developing as a critical practitioner. She also offers some thoughts on developing as a critical professional, which she suggests involves: developing emotional intelligence; knowing and using inner resources; challenging, exercising self control and resisting pressure.

Table 3.1
Aspects of criticality

Critical questioning involves: • fundamental questions that explore what you know; • connecting questions that relate different perspectives; • hypothesis questions that move you on to considering a new perspective; • critical questions that involve creating and defending an argument.	*Critical reasoning* involves: • being aware of, and identifying, possible 'assumptions, bias and hidden agendas'.
Critical reading interrogates texts by asking: • who is the intended audience? • what are the claims made by the author? • how well does the argument work? • is the evidence valid?	*Critical writing* uses skills such as: • putting forward a main idea and clarifying assertions; • demonstrating an appreciation of the language used in an argument and responding to it; • being aware of the strengths and weaknesses of the argument being made; • assessing the logic and coherence of the argument and the validity of the material on which it is based.

Source: Drawing from Jones 2009: 8, 37, 57–8, 89

Transfer of learning

On entering a social work course, students are invited to consider how their past experiences – academic, personal and work-related – can assist them in developing their knowledge, skills and value base to become a professionally qualified social worker. At its simplest, transfer of learning occurs when prior learning affects new learning. Macaulay argues that transfer of learning is 'a subconscious process [which] occurs continuously'; however, conscious transfer in education and work is more complex (Macaulay 2000: 11). By making links between previous and present experiences your learning is enhanced. She describes how transfer can be *near*, where learning is transferred to a very similar situation, or *far*, in which learning is transferred to a very different situation. It is this latter form of transfer which is most relevant to social work. Students are required to transfer learning from the classroom to assist their work in practice, and to transfer learning in one practical situation with one service user group to another very different situation or service user group. Transfer of learning can also be *positive* in that the learning that is transferred to a new situation increases understanding, or *negative* in that the learning transferred is not used appropriately, in that it is unhelpful action or mistaken beliefs which are transferred. In order for positive, useful and appropriate transfer to occur, you need to be able to abstract general principles from a situation, using the skills of reflection and critical analysis discussed in the previous chapter, to assist the analysis of a new situation.

Everyday, fragmented and fluent approaches to transfer of learning

In her research with social work students and the integration of theory and practice, Secker (1993) found that three different approaches to transfer can be identified: *everyday*, *fragmented* and *fluent*.

An *everyday* approach is characterised as one in which 'the student [does] not draw on the kind of knowledge which is usually described as theoretical. Instead they [draw] solely on knowledge from their personal, everyday lives' (Secker 1993: 169). Cree (2000) suggests that this approach can lead to students treating service users as friends or family. I have provided an example of this based on my work as a tutor (Green Lister 2000). I explain how a student, at a placement/practice learning visit with the student, myself and the practice teacher, described a group session with parents who had children with learning disabilities, in which she was being directly observed by her practice teacher. In the meeting one mother described how she had difficulties caring for her thirteen-year-old son with learning disabilities, who was threatening to leave home. She stated that she had responded by sending her son into the back yard in his underclothes for a period of time. The student responded by describing her own experience with her daughter, whom she had allowed to leave the house with a suitcase and who was away from the home for a period of hours. The student had responded in a humorous, friendly and sympathetic way, but had not listened closely to the parent who had described a serious child care issue. When this was raised with the student she analysed that she had confused identification with empathy, and having been given positive feedback about her open approach on a previous occasion, had decided to 'act naturally'. On reflection, this student identified an inappropriate transfer of previous experience.

A *fragmented* approach taken by students in the transfer of learning is one in which students face dilemmas in practice as a result of conflict between everyday and theoretical knowledge, and are self-conscious about their theoretical justification of actions (Secker 1993). An example of this can be seen in a student's assessment of a young man, living with a female lone parent, who was engaging in troublesome behaviour. The student recommended that the young man be allocated a male social worker as he lacked a father figure. The student explained that this assessment was based on previous experiences of a member of her family, a recent television programme and her understanding of adolescent development. This student demonstrated 'an uncritical and haphazard' transfer of learning (Green Lister 2000: 171).

A *fluent* approach is one in which students make use of 'ready made theory in constructing their own theories' (Secker 1993: 78). An example of this approach was demonstrated by a student on placement working with a male drug user in prison. This student described how she had used her knowledge of feminist theory to understand the young man's disadvantaged position of living in poverty with poor educational achievements. As an adoptive parent, she also reflected on attachment theory to assist her understanding of the impact of the young man's experience of a number of separations in his childhood. She had exemplified *positive* and *far* transfer of learning.

Transfer of learning: contexts

Having given examples of successful and unsuccessful transfer of learning, the learning and teaching processes which assist transfer of learning will be discussed.

Positive transfer of learning needs to be supported in the learning context, either in the university or in practice. In the university, a learning and teaching approach is required that is based on the principles of adult learning and student-centred learning, which results in an open learning culture. Learning opportunities suitable to the academic stage of the student need to be provided. Some learning and teaching methods such as problem-based learning – which requires you to identify what it is you need to know, how you will find it, and then how this applies to the problem/situation – can assist this process. As you repeat this process over the period of a course, you are given the opportunity to transfer both skills and knowledge to different areas of the social work curriculum. In a study of mature students entering social work education (Green Lister 2003), students identified that being introduced to foundational theories and values at the start of a course provided a solid base for transfer of learning. Lecturers modelling the process of transfer by providing good examples were valued highly. Students in this study also found it useful for lecturers to be clear about the theoretical position/s from which they were teaching. The study found that:

> Students made particular mention of feminism and anti-oppressive frameworks which were described by one student as 'the glue that made everything hang together' and by another as 'the blue sky in the jigsaw'. Students explained that the use of these frameworks assisted them in distilling the essentials for their experience and making connections with new situations.
>
> (Green Lister 2003: 134)

These students also found that the recognition and valuing of their previous experience by lecturers and practice assessors enhanced their ability to use this as a basis for transfer. So exercises which encouraged students to reflect on and share experiences in a structured way were welcomed. However, as seen in the above example of a fragmented approach to learning transfer, making use of previous experience can be difficult. This study found that:

> When introduced to new concepts, or challenged on beliefs or assumptions, students can feel deskilled and find it hard to look at past experience positively. The very process of making connections can be painful as students interrogate their previous work practices. One student in the study who had extensive experience in child care work in both residential and fieldwork settings described how 'very emotional' she felt when being introduced to new material which she felt she could have used in her previous practice.
>
> (Green Lister 2003: 135)

As discussed in Chapter 2, the assessment strategies and tools in a course can significantly affect your approach to learning. Cree (2000) argues that the following criteria should be used to assess transfer of learning:

1. Being an active learner: seeking out knowledge and learning;

2. Being able to reflect on previous experience and knowledge;

3. Being able to see patterns and to make relevant connections between different experiences and sources of knowledge;

4. Being open and flexible, able to compare and discriminate critically;

5. Being able to use abstract principles appropriately;

6. Being able to integrate personal knowledge and experience with professional knowledge and experience.

(Cree 2000: 43)

So, the learning environment and learning and teaching practices in the academic environment should give you the opportunity to demonstrate learning transfer. The learning opportunities provided on placement are also required to be conducive to the demonstration of transfer of learning from both previous personal and university experience and different practice learning contexts.

Transfer of learning: diversity of student experience

While the transfer of learning by students is likely to entail elements of the processes outlined above, each student has unique experiences which will mean that the learning process varies from person to person. The following vignettes are examples of students' pathways into social work education, and the activities that follow draw on them. Note that *different kinds* of information are provided in each vignette.

VIGNETTES

Parveen

Parveen is eighteen years old. She is a Muslim. She has entered the social work degree as a school leaver. She studied social science-based courses at her school and gained Bs and Cs in her subjects. She volunteered in a play scheme over two summers, and is working part time as a befriender during the social work course. Her parents both work in the health service. In school she was involved in a number of societies including drama and music.

John

John is forty-two years old. He entered the social work programme as a mature student. He left school at the age of sixteen and worked in industry for twenty years before being made redundant. John volunteered in a local day centre for people with learning disabilities before being employed as a care worker. He worked as a care worker for several years before deciding he would like to work as a qualified worker. John has a partner and two children in their teens.

Sonja

Sonja is thirty-five years old. She is white and does not follow a religion. Sonja is a lone parent of two small children. Sonja left school with some qualifications and worked in secretarial positions. After the birth of her two children she returned to education and undertook an access course. She has been assessed as having dyslexia. Her course involved placements in the care sector in residential homes. She is a member of her local community centre and is involved in organising a range of community events.

Kenneth

Kenneth is twenty-five years old. He lives with his male partner. He previously started a degree course in history on leaving school. After one year he decided to leave the course. He then worked for several years in a bar before travelling to Thailand, Vietnam, and then Malawi. During that time he became involved in working with local community groups and is now an active member of an international aid organisation.

At various stages in a social work course such as induction, prior to each practice learning experience and on leaving the course, students are asked to identify their learning needs since this is an important aspect of becoming an active and adult learner. For many students it is straightforward to identify specific knowledge they require but less straightforward to identify needs around the development of critical and reflective skills and the transfer of learning. The exercise at the end of this chapter provides a useful basis for this process.

Exercise 1: Factors affecting transfer of learning in the vignettes

Factors such as age, place of birth, ethnic background, sexuality, family background, academic qualifications, work experience and religious beliefs may all influence the way in which transfer of learning takes place. However, it is important not to make assumptions about the impact, for example, of age or religious beliefs. The following questions are prompts for you to consider with regard to each person described above. Again, note that not all information is provided about each person.

Personal characteristics

- What personal characteristics are known?

- What personal characteristics are unknown?

- What impact *might* the known and unknown characteristics (e.g. age, ethnicity, sexuality, religious beliefs, political beliefs) have on the student's ways of transferring learning? Why might these factors have an impact?

Family background/current living situation

- What is known about the family background/current living situation?

- What impact *might* the known and unknown characteristics (e.g. life experience, living situation, support/commitments) have on the student's ways of transferring learning?

- Why might these factors have an impact?

Academic background

- What is known about their academic experience?

- What is unknown?

- Does it appear to be relevant to a social work course?

- What makes it relevant? The subject area? Level of qualification? Other?

- How much are academic qualifications an indicator of academic ability?

- What other factors impact on academic ability?

- What impact *might* the known and unknown characteristics have on transfer of learning?

- Why might these factors have an impact?

Work experience background

- What is known about the work experience background?

- What is unknown?

- What impact might the known and unknown work experience (e.g. type of experience, length of experience, paid or unpaid, location of experience) have on the student's ways of transferring learning?

- Why might these factors have an impact?

> **Exercise 2: Factors affecting your own transfer of learning**
>
> Having considered the factors which may influence the people represented in the vignettes, now use the framework to consider what factors might influence your own transfer of learning.

Key learning points

- Reflection is the process of looking back and considering what, why and how a situation developed and how that might have changed.

- Criticality involves the skills of observation, exploring and questioning. It requires consideration of the different perspectives from which a situation might be seen.

- Transfer of learning may be everyday, fragmented or fluent. Fluency requires students to see patterns and connections which may assist understanding, but avoids an unthinking transfer of these to a new situation.

Further reading

Jones, S. (2009) *Critical learning for social work students*, Exeter: Learning Matters.

Walker, H. (2008) *Studying for your social work degree*, Exeter: Learning Matters.

4 Theoretical explanations
How and where to look

When asked to apply theory to practice, you may find it difficult to navigate through the plethora of theoretical texts to identify the theories which are most relevant to your work, whether that be an academic assignment or a piece of work in practice. In this chapter you will be taken through the *process* of considering what theoretical material would be pertinent to developing an understanding of an academic or practice scenario.

First, you will be introduced to the key principles of inquiry used in research, based on guidance drawn from the research literature. An academic scenario will be used to exemplify how the research process can assist you with regard to *how* and *where* to look for theoretical explanations when undertaking academic assignments. This process can equally be applied to practice situations but, in order to give students a choice of approaches, another inquiry process will be introduced here for these.

So, in the second section of this chapter, problem-based learning (PBL), briefly explained in Chapter 2, will be described and applied to a practice situation. PBL is a method of inquiry that can usefully be adapted to provide a framework showing how and where to look for theoretical explanations and supporting knowledge, when working in a practice situation.

A research process applied to answering academic assignments: an overview

Stage 1: Identifying the key research questions, aims or goals

At the start of any research process, the core task is to identify the key questions that need to be answered. This involves anticipating the end of the research process and reflecting on what needs to be known by the end of this process. After generating a number of possibilities, the aim of identifying research questions is to clarify the purpose of the research activity. The key research questions assist you to be clear about your final goal. Another way of describing this initial process is defining your aim or your goal. The importance of this stage is to ensure that you have clarity of purpose in your information gathering.

So, when given an academic assignment you need to identify specifically what the assignment requires you to do and then what your research questions are, for the purpose of knowing *how* and *where* to look for theory. A useful way of starting this is by identifying key words and then framing research questions, which will assist you to find the appropriate theoretical explanations.

Useful ways of framing research questions are:

1. How far, and in what ways, are the needs of older people met in community-based services?

2. What evidence is there of inter-professional working in the assessment of young people with learning disabilities?

3. What are the views and experiences of survivors of domestic abuse of social work services?

4. To what extent are young people's views of the child protection system taken into account by professionals when designing policy?

5. What explanations are there for high re-offending rates among young people on probation?

Stage 2: Developing research objectives

Answering the research questions requires you to identify those objectives that will assist you to achieve your final goal. Objectives can be defined as stepping stones or mini goals.

The following example phrases are useful ways of formulating objectives (and see later in the chapter for a full example of an assignment with its objectives and goal). Note that the emphasis is on what you will *do*.

'The objective of this research is . . . :

*   to ascertain . . . ';

*   to discover . . . ';

- to identify . . . ';

- to explore . . . ';

- to draw out . . . ';

- to define . . . ';

- to describe . . . ';

- to illustrate . . . ';

- to analyse . . . ';

- to compare . . . .'

In order to establish objectives, it is useful to identify key words or phrases to establish a basis for searching for information. At this stage the emphasis is on *clarifying* the question and *identifying* the information that needs to be gathered. It is important not to make assumptions and there is no rush to jump to conclusions.

Stage 3: Systematic data collection, and where to start looking for theoretical approaches

Textbooks

A starting point for many of you in seeking to access theory is to turn first of all to social work textbooks, which you may have been directed to in your course or module reading lists or which have been recommended by lecturers or practice assessors/teachers. Textbooks are an extremely useful resource. Some texts, like this one, are introductions aimed at social work students towards the start of their course. Others –for example Coulshed and Orme (2006), Fook (2002), and Payne (2005) – are broadly aimed at students at a later stage in their social work education.

Crisp *et al.* (2006) discuss the uses and limitations of textbooks as a source of information for students. Textbooks which are current are a good source of information with regard to current debates in the subject as they provide information on the core areas which the profession deems important to understand.

However, it is important that textbooks are up to date and comprehensively cover the areas they purport to discuss, as they are very influential in determining what students believe they should know. Crisp *et al.* (2006) argue that introductory sociology textbooks, for example, *socialise* or *acculture* students into the discipline. That is, the content of textbooks, the theories they emphasise and the ethic or values they promote, send strong messages to students about the nature of knowledge, and what it is they need to know. If the author favours a particular theoretical stance, you may find that the text only discusses that stance and omits other significant approaches, so you receive only a partial under-standing of the entirety of the subject area. There is also concern that textbooks may try to be too comprehensive and so offer a superficial consideration of the subject – a process which is called 'mentioning'. Finally, in their review of textbooks, Crisp *et al.* (2005, 2006) found that the books tended to be located in Western culture and paid little attention to diversity across cultures, class and gender. This could encourage students to accept the current social order rather than see it as their role to challenge it. As Cherlin (1997) argues, 'What matters most in a textbook is whether or not it stimulates critical thought. That cannot be done by telling students the correct answers because, far more often than we would like to admit, there are no correct answers' (Cherlin 1997: 210). Ornstein (1994) suggests that, when considering recommending a textbook, social work educators should consider the following criteria. It is also useful for you as a student to bear these questions in mind:

- Is the text up to date and accurate?

- Is it comprehensive?

- Does it adequately and properly portray minority ethnic communities and women?

- Are the objectives, headings and summaries clear?

- Are the contents and index well organised?

- Is it durable enough to last several years?

- What are the outstanding features of the text?

- What are the shortcomings of the text?

- Do the outstanding features strongly override the shortcomings?

(Ornstein 1994: 71–2)

Electronic search of databases
Generic databases like Google Scholar are useful starting points to get an idea of the range of literature which is available. However a basic search can generate thousands of references and it is time-consuming to filter these. There are a number of social science databases which can be searched from the university library catalogue. A useful one, for example, which contains within it a number of data bases is Cambridge Scientific Abstracts. This database provides a useful tutorial on how to undertake an initial search and then how to refine your search.

Electronic search of key journals
A third search strategy is to identify key journals and search within them with key terms or key authors. This provides a more focused search. There are some key journals such as the *British Journal of Social Work* which cover a large range of topics. Others are more specific to a subject or service user group. University libraries provide facilities to search for relevant journals using key words. Examples of subject topics and related journals are:

Table 4.1
Key subject-specific journals

Subject topic	Journals
Child abuse and child protection	*Child Abuse Review*
	Children and Society
Learning disability	*British Journal of Learning Disability*
	Disability and Society
Offending behaviour	*Probation*
	British Journal of Criminology
Learning and teaching in social work	*Social Work Education*

Relevant websites

Finally, it is useful to search relevant websites for material which is termed 'grey' or unpublished. Social work educators usually advise caution to students with regard to broad searches on the web as this can result in access to websites which do not always have academically rigorous content. However, judicious searches of websites of, for example, voluntary organisations can lead to the unearthing of useful material such as research reports, briefing papers, service user views and practice guides. At this stage ensure that you keep an accurate and complete list of references that you have viewed and rejected, or viewed and read, to avoid repetition of work.

Stage 4: Data analysis

Having gathered a range of data, your task will then be to sift through to identify the most relevant journal articles and texts.

Review the objectives

Using your objectives as a checklist will ensure that you have covered all the areas that you set out to. At this stage, returning to your key words is useful in helping you to do this. Practical techniques such as reading abstracts of articles, and chapter summaries will assist the process.

Chapter 3

Return to the guidelines for critical analysis
To assist your analysis it is useful to return to the guidelines for developing critical analysis provided in Chapter 3:

- Ensure you have grasped the key information/arguments.

- Ascertain the basis of the argument – the theoretical/research evidence.

- Question the evidence.

- Explore the merits or constraints of each argument, considering, for example, value base, research evidence, and the coherence of the argument.

Theoretical explanations

- Compare the different arguments.

- Make a judgement as to what your opinion is and ensure you have evidence to justify it.

- Acknowledge the possible critiques of your own judgement.

- Draw a conclusion.

Stage 5: Writing up

Having mapped out your responses to your objectives and engaged in the process of critical analysis, you can then return to your research questions in order to answer the assignment question.

At this stage it is important not to underestimate the length of time it takes to write an assignment. Very often in the process of writing up you may find you need to return to the original data, and your initial conclusions may be challenged as you develop your argument. Healy and Mulholland's (2007) text on writing skills for social workers provides very comprehensive guidance on a range of forms of writing required in social work education and social work. In the first chapter of their book they offer advice on how to design a document which could be applied to student social work assignments.

This outline of the research process will now be applied to an academic scenario which is an example of an assignment question for students on the first year of their degree in social work.

ACADEMIC SCENARIO

Consider the following academic assignment.

Year 1 assessment task (Module: Children in society)

On the one hand it has been argued that the adolescent years of children are 'storm and stress' (Hall 1904). On the other it could be argued that this notion of adolescence is outdated though still influential in how young people in their teenage years are viewed. This view suggests that adolescent behaviour is not exceptional and young people are labelled by society.

Give reasons for why each view may or may not be helpful in understanding young people's behaviour.

Conclude with your own opinion, giving the reason for this opinion.

Stage 1: Identifying the key research questions, aims or goals

- What evidence is there to support the two theoretical approaches of *storm and stress* and *labelling* to explain young people's behaviour?

- What conclusions do I draw and why?

Stage 2: Establishing objectives

Identification of key words

In this assignment question the key words which refer to theoretical explanations are:

- *adolescent*;

- *storm and stress*;

- *labelling*.

Objectives

- to find the text from which the quotation is taken;

- to identify who the key writers are in the field of adolescent development;

- to explain the key theoretical understandings of adolescent development;

- to explore the arguments of those who support the 'storm and stress' theory;

- to explore the critiques of the theory;

- to define labelling;

- to identify the key arguments by authors who theorise about labelling;

- to analyse and compare the arguments made in both approaches;

- to make a judgement on their validity and to form a reasoned opinion.

Stage 3: Systematic data collection

Textbooks

(Checklist: date; accuracy; comprehensiveness; attention to black and minority ethnic people and to women; clear context and index; durability; outstanding features and shortcomings.)

With regard to the assignment question, one possible source textbook is Sigelman and Rider's 2009 text on human development and the life span. An initial scan of this text indicates that it is recent, published in 2009, and significant and durable as it is in its sixth edition. The contents section indicates that it is very comprehensive, which is the outstanding feature. There is a specific section on culturally sensitive research. The contents and index are well organised and signpost where to find material. The outstanding aspect is that it encourages a critical approach, with a chapter devoted to an exploration of *how* development is studied, and then chapters devoted to summaries of different theories of adolescent development. The shortcoming of the text for this assignment question is that the section which specifically looks at adolescence is fairly short. So, on balance this would be a useful starter text from which to follow up further references.

Electronic search of databases
Initial Google Scholar search results:

- *adolescent development*   1,120,000

- *storm and stress*   294,000

- *labelling theory*   408,000

- *labelling theory adolescence*   25,000

A brief scan of the first few pages of results was useful in that it identified the source reference of the term 'storm and stress' (Hall 1904), and showed that there were significant critiques of the concept. A range of writers on adolescent labelling emerged and this is useful information to assist refining terms in a search of other databases.

Initial search of *Cambridge Scientific Abstracts*
An introductory quick search in the area of Social Sciences, of publications from 2005 of adolescent development, revealed 2,505 publications including journals, peer-reviewed journals, conferences and books.

Electronic search of key journals
The third search strategy of identifying key journals to provide a more focused search strategy could concentrate on the journals of *Child Development*, *Child Development Perspectives* or *New Directions in Child and Adolescent Development.*

Relevant websites
A relevant website for this research question is the National Children's Bureau, where there is useful material on young people's views of violence.

Stage 4: Data analysis

Review the objectives
Objectives:

- to find the text from which the quotation is taken;

- to identify who the key writers are in the field of adolescent development;

- to explain the key theoretical understandings of adolescent development;

- to explore the arguments of those who support the 'storm and stress' theory;

- to explore the critiques of the theory;

- to define labelling;

- to identify the key arguments by authors who theorise about labelling;

- to analyse and compare the arguments made in both approaches;

- to make a judgement on their validity and to form a reasoned opinion.

Your literature search will have equipped you with the core material with which to meet the first seven objectives. To reach these objectives is a matter of summarising the literature pertinent to each objective. Inevitably there will be an element of description to this. You will need to rehearse *what* the theorists are saying.

Return to the guidelines for critical analysis
- Ensure you have grasped the key information/arguments.

- Ascertain the basis of the argument – the theoretical/research evidence.

- Question the evidence.

- Explore the merits or constraints of each argument, considering, for example, value base, research evidence, and the coherence of the argument.

- Compare the different arguments.

The final three objectives require you to use your skills of critical analysis. The final stages in developing a critically analytical answer are:

- Make a judgement as to what your opinion is, ensuring you have evidence to justify it.

- Acknowledge the possible critiques of your own judgement.

- Draw a conclusion.

Stage 5: Writing up

Having mapped out responses to objectives and engaged in the process of critical analysis, now return to the research questions in order to answer the assignment question.

What evidence is there to support the two theoretical approaches of *storm and stress* and *labelling* to explain young people's behaviour?

What conclusions do I draw and why?

An adapted problem-based learning process applied to a practice scenario

Problem-based learning (PBL) as a learning strategy was developed initially in medicine at McMaster University, Ontario in the 1960s. Variations of PBL such as Enquiry and Action Learning (EAL) or Enquiry-based Learning (EBL) have similar characteristics. PBL is an approach to learning used within social work education and other areas to assist students to become self-directed learners. PBL encourages students to learn though a structured exploration of a research problem. Typically, students work in small groups and are given a practice scenario to explore. To be effective in PBL, students need to develop skills of independent learning, problem identification, problem solving and, in most cases, team work. In group-based PBL students discuss the problem, share existing knowledge and identify gaps, and identify areas of exploration from which tasks for exploration are allocated to group members. Following the completion of tasks the PBL group then reconvenes to share and discuss the learning.

Boud and Feletti (2007), in reviewing the research evidence on the efficacy of PBL, argue that the benefits of PBL lie in the fact that as a learning process it takes into account how students actually learned through being actively involved in their learning. They suggest that as a learning tool in the university the practice base element of PBL scenarios means it is professionally relevant. The rate of the growth of knowledge in any particular professional field means that a curriculum cannot fit everything into conventional lectures. The problems with the use of the approach they find, for students, are that the process of PBL might develop into the routine activity of problem solving rather than wider problem exploration. Furthermore, students who are used to more traditional approaches may find the process confusing or stressful.

The process of PBL

The following seven stages are typical of the process of PBL. The time scales between these stages would be determined by the practice or academic context. For example, in university, the information-gathering stage may range from a number of hours, if the PBL takes a day workshop format, or a week, if a group meets once a week. If you are undertaking PBL in practice learning, the time scales may be determined by you, taking into account agency deadlines, or by a practice supervisor who may wish you to undertake the PBL process in between supervision sessions.

In the example below, which shows how PBL can assist in looking for theoretical explanations and supporting knowledge, the element of team work is not developed. Rather, the PBL approach is adapted to provide tools which will enable you to explore a case scenario and to develop skills in how and where to look for theoretical explanations and supporting knowledge. In this adapted approach, the PBL process is presented as a single seven-stage process that individual students can use when presented with a practice scenario. Clearly, this process can be repeated as new issues emerge in the scenario.

Stage 1: Presentation of practice scenario
In Stage 1 the student is presented with a practice scenario. Typically, brief information will be provided to allow you to explore a range of issues, rather than focus on a particular route of problem solution. The aim of the practice scenario is to *open up* areas of exploration and investigation.

Stage 2: Trigger
The *trigger* is presented to the student at Stage 2. The trigger is a statement or piece of information which activates the process of problem investigation. It opens up debate and serves as a prompt as to the area you will need to explore. Some examples of triggers are:

- a quotation from one of the people introduced in the scenario;

- a new piece of information such as a letter from a general practitioner or phone call from a neighbour;

- a citation from a book;

- a clip from a newspaper article;

- notification of a new event;

- copy of recent correspondence;

- a video clip.

Stage 3: Identification of possible problems
In this stage the practice scenario and the trigger are explored. The emphasis is on determining:

- What is known about the situation?

- What possible problems or issues might emerge from the situation and require future exploration?

A brief statement of potential issues is drawn together.

Stage 4: Preliminary analysis of the problems/hypothesising

Having listed the potential issues, the next stage is to engage in a preliminary analysis of these issues. This stage is also called *hypothesising*. Hypothesising involves making tentative suggestions with regard to:

- What might be going on?

- What might be the potential explanations?

- What might be possible causes?

Stage 5: Research aims

At Stage 5 the areas which need to be researched are identified. Having considered possible issues, it is then important to consider:

- What do I know about this area, from academic study, practice or previous experience?

- What is not known; what are the gaps in my knowledge?

- What are the key areas for exploration?

- Where can I find information – be that theoretical explanations or supporting knowledge – that will assist me to address those gaps and increase my understanding?

Stage 6: Research

At Stage 6 *research action* takes place:

- research of the literature identified as requiring exploration, using the research process identified in the first half of the chapter – systematic data collection;

- practical research in terms of agency policy and practice, speaking to colleagues and other agencies about local resources, for example:

  - legal frameworks;

  - agency policies and procedures;

  - social work colleagues;

  - other professionals;

  - other agencies;

  - service user and carer groups.

Stage 7: Synthesis

The process of synthesising information is similar to that of data analysis in the research approach. Clearly, a review of all the literature is very time-consuming and would be an ongoing process. Discussions with other professionals and agencies will also need to be planned over time. By Stage 7, individual students using a PBL approach would need to be aware of the key theoretical explanations and key areas of supporting knowledge. These should be presented in a systematic way with future areas of investigation noted.

PRACTICE SCENARIO

Consider the following practice:

Stage 1: Presentation of practice scenario

Ruth is a lone parent. She has three children under the age of five, is unemployed and in debt to a number of agencies. She has been referred to the social worker by her General Practitioner, who has prescribed antidepressants for Ruth but considers that she needs a range of social supports.

Stage 2: Trigger

The case is allocated to a student social worker. Ruth speaks to the student social worker for the first time on the phone and states that she 'can't go on like this'. The student social worker has arranged to meet Ruth the following week. The practice teacher/assessor asks the student to come to the next supervision session having explored Ruth's situation in order to prepare for their first meeting with her.

Stage 3: Identification of possible problems

- What is known about the situation?

- What possible problems or issues might emerge from the situation and require future exploration?

Brief listing of potential issues:

- lone parenthood;

- depression;

- finance;

- children's needs;

- professional roles.

Stage 4: Preliminary analysis of the problems/hypothesising

- What might be going on for Ruth and her family?

- What might be the potential explanations for Ruth's depression and financial difficulties?

- What might be the possible causes of Ruth's problems?

Lone parenthood

In and of itself, lone parenthood is not a problem, however lone parenthood may be associated with:

- stress of sole responsibility of parenting;

- lack of social supports.

Depression

Ruth has sought and received medical treatment for depression; what links are there between this and her social situation?

Finance

Ruth has identified finance as an issue; again this may be linked to her status as a lone parent.

Children's needs

What, if any, impact has Ruth's situation on her children?

Professional roles

- What is the role of the social worker?

- What is the role of the GP?

- What are the roles of other professionals?

Stage 5: Research aims

- What do I know about lone parenthood and depression, from academic study, practice or previous experience?

- What is not known; what are the gaps in my knowledge?

- What are the key areas for exploration?

- Where can I find information – be that theoretical explanations or supporting knowledge – that will assist me to address those gaps and increase my understanding?

The following theoretical and supporting knowledge areas require investigation:

Lone parenthood:

- sociological literature on lone parenthood;

- incidence and prevalence;

- sociological explanations of impact – stigma, labelling, social isolation;

- gender issues in lone parenthood;

- black and minority ethnic issues in lone parenthood;

- parenting issues for lone parents;

- UK social policy on lone parenthood;

- UK-wide and specific country policies;

- local resources for lone parents.

Finance:

- social policy literature on poverty and lone parenthood;

- benefits and allowances for lone parents.

Children's needs:

At this stage it is not known if or how Ruth's situation has affected the children. Neither Ruth nor the GP have identified the children's needs as an issue. This might be an area for future exploration.

Professional roles:

- What is the role of the social worker?

- social work literature on assessment;

- social work literature on working with lone parents;

- social work literature on working with people with depression.

- What is the role of the GP?

- What are the roles of other professionals?

- At this stage these questions could be addressed by seeking advice from colleagues. The current focus is on gathering information to prepare for meeting with Ruth.

Stage 6: Research

- Research of the literature identified above using the research process identified in the first half of the chapter.

Key words: *lone parenthood*; *depression*.

- Practical research in terms of agency policy and practice, speaking to colleagues and other agencies about local resources:

  - legal frameworks – supporting children and families, benefit legislation;

  - agency policies and procedures – assessment procedures and time scales;

  - social work colleagues with experience in children and family and mental health work;

  - other professionals – GP, health visitor, district nurse;

  - other agencies – voluntary agencies working with lone parents, childcare organisations;

  - service user and carer groups – lone parent support groups.

Stage 7: Synthesis

As noted above, exploration of all the identified literature would be very time-consuming, and is a longer-term project. When you start the process of assessment, some issues are likely to emerge as priorities, and these are the ones which require more in-depth exploration.

In preparation for the supervision, you prepare a report which outlines the stages of the investigation as detailed above. In the report you would:

- identify the issues that require investigation;

- provide a summary of the initial findings from the literature on the issues identified above;

- outline the intended process of investigation;

- list literature/resources already identified;

- provide a summary of information gleaned from colleagues and other agencies.

In this chapter we have offered two approaches to assist students to know *how* and *where* to look for theoretical explanations and underpinning knowledge. A research approach was applied to answer an academic assignment and a PBL approach used to explore a practice scenario.

Exercise 1: Academic scenario

> Social exclusion is a process. It can involve the systematic denial of entitlements to resources and services, and the denial of the right to participate on equal terms in social relationships in economic, social, cultural or political arenas.
>
> (Governance and Social Development Resource Centre, n.d.)

Discuss in relation to one socially excluded group.

Use Stages 1 and 2 of the research process, summarised below, to plan how you would begin to answer this question.

- Identify the research questions, aims or goals.

- Develop research objectives.

- Begin systematic data collection.

    - Identify one core textbook – does it meet Ornstein's (1994) criteria?

    - Identify one electronic database.

- Using your key words, practise searching the database for material which would assist you to answer your research question.

- Identify one relevant organisation, visit the website and identify useful publications.

Exercise 2: Practice scenario

A practice scenario (Stage 1) and a trigger (Stage 2) are presented below. Using Stages 3 to 5 of the PBL process, consider how you would approach preparing for meeting David, who is allocated to you on his release from hospital. Although a Community Care assessment was undertaken by the social worker located in the hospital, it is important that you are prepared with regard to the issues that David may present. Consider what theoretical explanations and supporting knowledge you would require to prepare for your contact with David.

Stage 1: Presentation of practice scenario

David has been in hospital for a hip replacement. David is seventy years old and lives alone. The social worker based in the hospital has assessed David's needs on discharge. A Community Care assessment has been made and a plan has been constructed by the hospital social worker.

Stage 2: Trigger

On discharge, a community-based social work agency is contacted and David is allocated a worker from this team. You are the allocated worker.

Stage 3: Identification of possible problems

- What is known about David's situation?

- What possible problems or issues might emerge from David's situation which require future exploration?

- Statement of potential issues.

Stage 4: Preliminary analysis of the problems/hypothesising

- What might be going on for David?

- What might be the potential explanations?

- What might be possible causes?

Stage 5: Research aims

- What do I know about community care and discharge from hospital, from academic study, practice or previous experience?

- What is not known; what are the gaps in my knowledge?

- What are the key areas for exploration?

- Where can I find information – be that theoretical explanations or supporting knowledge – that will assist me to address those gaps and increase my understanding?

Key learning points

- A systematic approach to knowing how and where to look for theory can be developed using a research process and a PBL process.

- Identifying relevant theories involves an organised search across a range of sources.

- This approach can be applied to both academic and practice situations.

Further reading

Boud, D. and Feletti, G. (eds) (1997) *The challenge of problem-based learning*, 2nd edn, London: Kogan-Page, pp. 1–14.

Healey, K. and Mulholland, J. (2002) *Writing skills for social workers*, London: Sage.

5 Anti-oppressive theories and concepts

A key requirement in social work education is that students demonstrate anti-oppressive practice. This requirement can be daunting for many students because anti-oppressive practice is a broad term. It can also suggest that being anti-oppressive is all about *doing*. An essential aspect of anti-oppressive practice is also an understanding of the *theoretical* underpinnings of such practice. This chapter will introduce you to the various concepts which might constitute anti-oppressive practice. It is important to note that you will be provided with beginning definitions of these concepts, signposting you to key authors, and that you will need to explore the original texts in order to develop a deeper understanding of their meanings. In Chapter 6 we will examine the processes of anti-oppressive practice.

It is useful to see anti-oppressive theory as consisting of a range of different concepts and approaches. These concepts have their own distinct features but are also inter-related. It is useful to take a portfolio approach to using these concepts in building an understanding of anti-oppressive theory and practice. There are many areas which inform anti-oppressive practice. The elements of this chapter are:

• social divisions;

• identity;

- power;

- oppression;

- anti-oppressive ethics.

Social divisions

Social divisions are widely perceived differences between large groups of people, characterised by inequalities in power and access to material and cultural resources, both individually and collectively. These differences vary through time and space. They are often long-standing, but can sometimes alter quickly during periods of general social change. The key social divisions are usually considered as: class or position in the economic and social structure; race or ethnic background; gender; disability; age; and sexuality. Payne's (2006) text provides a comprehensive discussion of social divisions. There are other sources of inequality such as unemployment, culture, religion, language and mental health which contribute to oppression as well as to the processes of marginalisation in society. An overview of major approaches in social work to social divisions is provided below.

Radical approaches

The radical approaches to social work that developed in the 1970s (Bailey and Brake 1975; Corrigan and Leonard 1978; Langan and Lee 1989) are essentially concerned with class. These approaches are informed by Marxist analyses of capitalist society. These analyses see our society as fundamentally unequal as a result of the capitalist economic system, where one class, the bourgeoisie, owns private property and the other, the working class, provides the labour which produces the profit for the middle classes. This inherent economic inequality is thought to determine the operation of all other aspects of society including the political system, the family and religion. Marxist critique also states that the system is perpetuated by the working classes and the middle classes, who have been socialised into accepting this situation as a given, 'normal' and unchangeable state. A key Marxist concept is that of 'alienation'. This is a process by which workers have become operatives in a production line. Workers do not work to produce a finished product but rather perform just one aspect of the production process. Writing in the context of industry, working in a production line meant that workers could not communicate with other workers and did not see the finished product. As a result they became dehumanised and alienated from their work, other workers and themselves.

Radical social work writers understand social work as having complex and contradictory functions. On the one hand social work serves to ameliorate the worst aspects of capitalism by supporting the working class, or under-privileged. On the other hand social work supports the state by this very action, and so pacifies the oppressed. More recent approaches informed by Marxism explore how aspects of Marxist theory can assist both social workers and service users in critiquing social work structures and practice.

For example, Ferguson and Lavalette (2004) argue that the Marxist concept of 'alienation' can be used to understand the loss of control of social workers and the powerlessness of service users in contemporary social work practice. They argue that alienation theory can assist social workers and service users to understand social work structures and processes, and develop emancipatory social work practice.

Feminist approaches

Feminist approaches to social work are primarily concerned with the social construction of gender and the resulting gender inequalities in society. They are concerned with how gender identities are 'performed', that is, played out in social relationships and social structures. There are a wide range of feminist social work approaches which reflect different theoretical, political and practice concerns. Typically, the different feminist approaches have been characterised as liberal, radical, socialist, and postmodern approaches (see Payne 2005 for a succinct overview). Fook provides interesting reflections on her personal experience of different feminist approaches, and on structural approaches in general (Fook 2002: 5–14). Dominelli (2002: 162–63) argues that there are core feminist principles and characteristics relevant to social work practice:

- recognising the diversity of women;

- valuing women's strengths;

- eliminating the privileging of certain groups of women to prevent difference from becoming a basis for unequal power relations between different groups of women;

- considering women as active agents capable of making decisions for themselves in all aspects of their lives;

- locating individual women in their social situations and acknowledging the interconnectedness between the individual and collective entities relevant to them;

- providing women with the space to voice their own needs and solutions to problems;

- acknowledging the principle 'the personal is political' as relevant at macro, meso and micro levels of practice;

- redefining private woes as public issues;

- ensuring that women's needs are being addressed within the context of their being seen as whole human beings in which each area of life interacts with others;

- recognising the interdependent nature of human relations and, through that, realising that what happens to one individual or group has implications for everyone else;

- recognising that women's individual problems have social causes and addressing both levels in each intervention; and

- looking for collective solutions to individual problems.

Caution in taking an uncritical approach to feminist social work is advised by Orme (2003). She argues that students and social workers may take a simplistic stance towards feminist social work and that it is important to explore the theoretical differences within feminism in order to ensure critical practice. She cites debates between postmodern feminists and standpoint feminists' approaches to domestic violence. Standpoint feminists would perceive domestic violence from the perspective of the oppressed group, identified as women. Postmodern feminists would critique this approach as both 'homogenising' women, that is, not acknowledging differences between women, and also ignoring the voices of men, both perpetrators and victims, which they argue need to be heard to develop a critical understanding of domestic violence.

Anti-racist approaches and black perspectives

Anti-racist and black perspective approaches to social work developed during the 1980s and 1990s (Ahmad 1990; Dominelli 2008). Key features of black perspectives include recognition of different cultures and histories, valuing difference and promoting positive images of black people. Anti-racist social work aims to address racism at individual, cultural and structural levels.

There has been concern among some academics that anti-racist social work has been diluted in favour of a multi-cultural approach. For example, Heron (2004) argues that in contrast to a multi-cultural approach which he suggests aims to address mutual understandings and misunderstandings, 'the anti-racist perspective locates the problem in the fabric of British society' (Heron 2004: 227). His empirical work in the area found that '[t]he extent to which students are actually equipped to engage with "race" and discrimination is unclear' (p. 278).

Similarly, Graham (2009: 268) suggests that the 'dilution of anti-racist work into a discriminatory practice framework undermined the place of black perspectives in social work education'. She suggests that three key aspects need to be addressed to address different forms of marginalisation and exclusion from different perspectives:

> First, black perspectives can reclaim the histories, cultures, language and traditions and religions of black communities and understand their relevance to social work. Second, black perspectives can uncover and challenge the complex layers and varied mechanisms of oppression which contribute to contemporary forms of exclusion and marginalisation. Third, this approach can articulate the changing needs and priorities of black communities.
>
> (Graham 2009: 277–8)

The over-representation of black and minority ethnic children in residential care (Barn 1993; Kendrick 2008) and child protection proceedings (Chand and Thoburn 2006) and the historical neglect of the needs of black elders (Dominelli 2002) demonstrate that anti-racist social work remains an important area for students and practitioners to continue to develop. However, what is also clear is that black and minority ethnic families should not be seen as a homogeneous group and students need to be aware of diversities within communities.

Disability rights movements

During the 1990s a variety of disability movements emerged. Oliver and Sapey (1999) are two of the foremost proponents of the social model of disability, the basis of which is that it 'distinguishes between impairment and disability, the former referring to some form of physical loss, while the latter is taken as disadvantages, restrictions and oppression that occur as a result of social responses to impairment' (Sapey 2009: 336).

So, disability has been constructed through processes of labelling, segregating and focusing on individual impairments. Sapey (2009) challenges the assumption that disabled people necessarily require social work *care*, and argues that if social provisions were made, a disabled person would be no more likely to need assistance than a non-disabled person. In the field of learning disability, emphasis in social work practice has historically adopted a normalising approach. Normalisation theory 'is concerned with issues such as dress, the normal rhythms of people's day, the locations and company in which people spend their time and the things people spend their time doing' (Stainton 2009: 350). It has been criticised for being based on the assumption of what is 'normal' and 'desirable', and for focusing on the needs of individuals to change and adapt (Oliver 1990). The emphasis is now on adopting a rights-based and citizenship approach, which will be discussed in the next chapter.

Addressing ageism

Ageism has been defined as generating and reinforcing 'a fear and denigration of the ageing process, and stereotyping presumptions regarding competence and the need for protection' (Bytheway 1995: 14). It systematically denies resources and opportunities to a group of people based on their chronological age. Ageism has been constructed by economic structures, political values, cultural heritage, historical legacy and social attitudes (Tanner and Harris 2008: 12). Tanner and Harris (2008) summarise the values and principles which Hughes (1995) argues constitute anti-ageist practice.

The values of anti-ageist practice:

- personhood: recognising the equal value and status of every individual;

- citizenship: recognising that every individual is an equally important member of society with rights and responsibilities;

- celebration: according value to old age as a life phase and celebrating diversity among older people.

The principles of anti-ageist practice:

- empowerment: enabling older people to take control of their own lives;

- participation: facilitating the meaningful involvement of older people;

- choice: facilitating older people's ability to make choices and decisions;

- integration: working to integrate older people into mainstream activities, rather than segregating them;

- normalisation: making available whatever is needed to enable older people to continue living their lives as they want to.

(Tanner and Harris 2008: 17)

Tanner and Harris note 'some of the dangers and limitations of using "old age" as a social category' (2008: 21). On the one hand this can 'create and reaffirm ageist assumptions and practices', but on the other hand, by not specifically identifying old people, there is a 'danger of lapsing into "agelessness"', and so denying the changes that do take place over the life course (Tanner and Harris 2008: 21). Furthermore, Marshall *et al.* (2005: 33) argue, 'It is crucial to acknowledge the diversity in social, cultural, economic, financial, political, gender, generational and ethnic circumstances among others'.

Anti-heterosexist practices

Sexual orientation and sexual identity are both terms used to describe a person's sexual choice of or preference in a partner. A person's sexual orientation may be lesbian, gay, bisexual, asexual or heterosexual. In addition they may identify as transgender or transvestite. In the past twenty years social theorists have argued that sexual orientation is socially constructed, that is, influenced by the society and times we live in, rather than being determined *biologically* or *naturally*. Social work practice with gay and lesbian people has also been critiqued during this period (Cosis Brown 1998), as has social work education on the issue (Trotter and Gilchrist 1996). Jeyasingham (2008) argues that hetero-sexuality has been privileged in social work practice and resulted in a lack of awareness of issues faced by lesbians and gay men. Hafford-Letchfield (2010) argues that sexual orientation issues are also marginalised in social work education, and by implication this means that students' understanding of issues around sexual orientation in social work may require further development. Referring to Charnley and Langley (2007), Hafford-Letchfield advises that: 'Anti-heterosexist practice requires motivation and a willingness by both learners and its facilitators to engage in reflective learning in which conceptual, theoretical understanding can be achieved alongside the development of culturally sensitive practice skills' (2010: 255). Similarly, Cosis Brown and Cocker argue that social work research should include the experiences of lesbians and gay men and that qualifying and post-qualifying courses should ensure that social work students 'are equipped to work effectively with lesbians and gay men' (2011: 157).

Bywater and Jones (2007) provide best practice guidelines for social workers when working with issues of sexuality. They suggest that it is important to have a value base based on the declaration of sexual rights as made by the International Planned Parenthood Federation (IPPF 2008) and that it is essential to have an understanding of how sexuality is socially constructed and how social workers might influence this in their practice. Being aware of discrimination around sexuality, being comfortable with one's own sexuality, not making assumptions, establishing clear boundaries and keeping up to date with sexuality issues are some of the core values that they advocate.

Clearly the above social divisions are not mutually exclusive and, as we discuss in the next chapter, social work practice needs to consider how we work with a diverse range of people who are likely to belong to a number of disadvantaged groups. Before this the key concepts of identity and culture, power, oppression, and anti-oppressive ethics will be discussed.

Identity and culture

Fook (2002) argues that a person's identity is complex. She explores the postmodern idea of identity which argues that people have multiple, fluid and contradictory identities. Fook would argue that, just as our identities are complex, so are the processes of power. So, it would be simplistic to analyse power as something that one person has and another person has not. She uses the postmodern term 'false binary' to describe the artificial setting up of two opposites – in this case the powerful and the powerless. For example, a woman may be a senior manager in an office and be in a position of relational power over men. However, within that environment she might find herself subject to sexist remarks by men and in that respect feel oppressed. At home she may be in relational power in respect of her children, but if her children have behavioural problems, she may feel that she has no parental power. She cares for her mother and so another complex power relation exists. An understanding of one's identity is usually bound up in a view about one's culture.

Culture consists of a set of beliefs and practices. It creates perspectives on how to view society. This ranges from perspectives on wider social issues such as reasons for unemployment, to very specific social practices such as queuing for a bus. In any society there are many diverse cultures. It could be argued that a Western world viewpoint has viewed cultures as something that other groups, such as black and minority ethnic groups, have. However, cultures are present in all societies, and are evident from family practices through to state organisations. As Clifford and Burke (2009) emphasise, the process of oppression involves dominant cultures gradually acquiring the power to define what 'the norm' is and what is valued in that society. For example, with regard to professionals' responses to working with black and minority ethnic families, concern has been expressed about the over-pathologising of parents by professionals (Chand 2000). However more attention is paid in the literature to the concept of 'cultural relativism' among professionals working with black and minority ethnic families. This term refers to the processes through which workers make assumptions about cultural practices and accept, for example, a lower standard of care, as this is viewed as culturally acceptable in the family's community. Lord Laming (2003) makes reference to this approach in his report on the death of Victoria Climbié. The culturally relative approach, which can be evident across all aspects of social work practice and in which all cultures are seen as equal, can result in professionals working to a rule of optimism which fails to challenge practices and to recognise the existence of needs or abuse.

Power

Central to an understanding of anti-oppressive practice is the debate around the concept of power. Smith offers a way of understanding power as 'the capacity, held individually or collectively, to influence either groups or individuals (including oneself) in a given context' (Smith 2008: 23). He provides a useful way of beginning to understand the different ways in which power operates and suggests that an analysis of power needs, first of all, to acknowledge the different modes of power: '*personal, positional* and *relational*' (Smith 2008: 42). His argument is summarised below.

- *Personal* power: this relates to individual characteristics of people, for example age and gender. He illustrates personal power with an example of an older person with dementia, who wants to remain in her home, but appears under pressure to consider residential accommodation.

- *Positional* power: this relates to social position, for example in the workplace. Smith's example of personal power relates to power within the workplace and organisational status.

- *Relational* power: this relates to interactive relationships between individuals' power and that of groups. The example of power he provides is with regard to the changing nature of family relationships.

He also suggests that we need to understand power as *potential, possession, process* and *product* (Smith 2008: 23) as is summarised below.

- *Potential* power: this relates to the concept of empowerment (discussed below) and can be seen as a facilitative resource.

- *Possession* power: this relates to power as an 'attribute, held by an individual or a body, by virtue of certain characteristics' (Smith 2008: 28).

- *Process* power: this relates to power being seen as a continually changing phenomenon, depending on ever-changing interactions and circumstances.

- *Product* power: this relates to power being a product of dynamic change, for example as a result of a process of empowerment of a service user.

As we see from the above ways of understanding power, it is a complex concept. It cannot be viewed simply as something owned by one person, group or organisation and not owned by another, but instead as fluid, multidimensional and contextual. The following discussion of a definition of oppression will further explore the complexities of this area.

Oppression

Oppression includes both the exploitative exercise of power by individuals and groups over others, and the structuring of marginalisation and inequality into everyday routines and rules,

> through the continuing acquisition and maintenance of economic, political and cultural capital by dominant groups over a long period of time, reflecting the existence of major social divisions. Oppression therefore arises from inequalities of power that can be *both* stable and *fluid*, affected by situational changes in individual and group circumstances, and by people's responses to them.
>
> (Clifford and Burke 2009: 16)

This is a complex definition which requires further explanation.

The exploitative exercise of power by individuals and groups over others

This might be seen as the most common understanding of oppression in which one individual or group in a powerful position uses power to exploit another group or individual, for example an employing organisation over staff or an older child bullying a younger child. If we look at the definition of social divisions, we can see that the exploitative use of power may be through not only individual or unique acts but through the creation by social divisions of unequal power relations where particular groups have dominance over another.

the structuring of marginalisation and inequality into everyday routines and rules

This phrase emphasises that the oppression of social groups is not incidental but is *structured*, that is, a consequence of the way in which society is organised. In this way, the marginalisation and unequal treatment of certain groups is incorporated into everyday life. So, the high number of young black people unemployed in a certain area is a consequence of the wider social oppression, but the presence of young black unemployed people on the streets of a northern city in the UK during the day is seen as an everyday normality, as is the lack of presence of people with learning disability, for example in theatres and clubs.

> through the continuing acquisition and maintenance of economic, political and cultural capital by dominant groups over a long period of time, reflecting the existence of major social divisions.

The dominant position of some groups is as a result of gaining and keeping increased power over time. So, the unemployment of the black young people is not a feature of a particular town at a particular difficult time in the economy. It builds on the long-term oppression of black people over centuries but presents in a particular way in the twentieth-century UK context. The oppression does not only occur economically and politically but also culturally. Viewed simply this would mean that certain cultural practices, for example Rastafarianism, are not valued, but cultural oppression is a more complex process.

> Oppression therefore arises from inequalities of power that can be both stable and fluid, affected by situational changes in individual and group circumstances, and by people's responses to them.

The importance of this statement in understanding oppression is that there may be some power relations, which remain stable over time as a result of the long-term accumulation of power, to which Clifford and Burke (2009) previously referred. However, for example there may be large-scale political events which change the balance of power, so power relations are not static. Another more straight-forward example of a change in a power situation is that an employee may become an employer. However changes in power relations are usually more subtle, as people's identities are complex.

Anti-oppressive ethics

Ethical considerations are a further feature in the development of anti-oppressive practice. Clifford and Burke (2009) usefully draw together anti-oppressive theory and ethical concerns to define anti-oppressive ethics.

> Anti-oppressive ethics are approaches to guiding action in the light of recognition of inequalities and powerlessness damaging to the individual and collective freedom and welfare, especially in relation to groups and individuals marginalised through membership of dominated and diverse social divisions.
>
> (Clifford and Burke 2009: 6)

They argue that:

> The aim of anti-oppressive ethics is to provide guidance to oppose, minimise and/or overcome those aspects of human relationships that express and consolidate oppression. The point of adding the descriptive term 'anti-oppressive' to qualify 'ethics' is to emphasise individual behaviour as inseparable from the unequal, political and social contexts in which it occurs.
>
> (Clifford and Burke 2009: 16)

Clifford and Burke (2009) argue that an anti-oppressive approach to ethics accepts the postmodern concept that power is multiple and diverse but argue that anti-oppressive practice requires that there is an emphasis on addressing unequal power relationships.

Locating yourself in the discussion of oppression, power, culture and identity

In order to practise in an anti-oppressive way it is important for you to understand your own experiences and positions with regard to your identity, power and experiences of oppression. At the end of this chapter you will be asked to locate yourself in the discussion of oppression, power and identity. The following example relates to a social work student towards the start of her social work course.

- Write a short description of yourself in which you place yourself in one of the major social categories identified above.

- Identify where you think you are most and least powerful with regard to your personal power.

- Identify where you think you are most and least powerful with regard to your positional power.

- Identify the contradictions in these power positions. How would you describe your relational power?

- Are there any other forms of discrimination to which you think you are subject? Why?

- Use ten words to describe your identity and your culture.

Student social worker response:

- I am a black working-class woman. I am in my thirties so not young, middle-aged nor old. I am able bodied. I am heterosexual.

- I have personal power as I am viewed as intelligent. I am able to study. I am able to articulate my thoughts well. I don't feel I have personal power because I am not able to afford expensive clothes or hair cuts and I think this does affect the way that people see me. I don't make an immediate impression.

- I have positional power in my role as a mother. In my part-time work I am a supervisor so I have some positional power. I am a student on a course and I don't have positional power.

- Personally, it depends where I am and who I am with as to whether I feel personally powerful or powerless. I can be feeling confident at one point and feel people are listening to me and then one nasty comment and I feel all the power goes to that person. As I work part-time I can go into work and a decision I have made has been changed, or someone just doesn't do what I ask them and I can't force them, so it depends on the circumstances – who else is in, if someone is in a bad mood, if I have power or not.

- I am a single parent, live on a council estate, don't have a car and have a son who has dyslexia. I think there is a lot of discrimination against lone parents – getting pregnant to get a house and that sort of thing. Some people have views that everyone on a council estate is a scrounger. Public transport is terrible and expensive so I can't get to jobs that I would prefer to go to. People, even some teachers, don't understand dyslexia.

- Woman intelligent black mother student funny helpful loyal patient 'broke' [no money].

The student has clearly identified where she thinks she sits within the major social divisions. She has identified other aspects of her situation about which she thinks she is subject to discrimination. It can be seen that this student identifies herself as having some personal power mainly based on her intelligence but feels that her physical appearance, due to her non-expensive clothes, detracts from her personal power. This personal power also feels compromised when she is in receipt of 'nasty' comments. Her positional power in her work is contextual too, depending on the staff present and their reaction to her. Her chosen ten words go beyond describing her positional power and move to describing personal qualities.

This chapter has introduced you to the concepts which inform anti-oppressive practice.

Exercise 1

1. Write a short description of yourself in which you place yourself in one of the major social categories identified above.

2. Identify where you think you are most and least powerful with regard to your personal power.

3. Identify where you think you are most and least powerful with regard to your positional power.

4. Identify the contradictions in these power positions. How would you describe your relational power?

5. Are there any other forms of discrimination to which you think you are subject? Why?

6. Use ten words to describe your identity.

Exercise 2

In your own words write a short paragraph to explain the different understandings of the concept of power.

Which explanation is nearest to your own understanding?

How can you expand your understanding?

Key learning points

- In order to engage in anti-oppressive practice it is important to understand the concepts which constitute anti-oppressive theory.

- Power and oppression are complex concepts and are defined differently by different people coming from different perspectives.

- An understanding of the complexity of identity requires critical thinking and reflection.

Further reading

Clifford, D. and Burke, B. (2009) *Anti-oppressive ethics and values in social work*, Basingstoke: Palgrave Macmillan.

Smith, R. (2008) *Social work and power*, Basingstoke: Palgrave Macmillan.

6 Anti-oppressive processes

Having considered the core theoretical concepts of anti-oppressive practice in the last chapter, this chapter will discuss the processes which can constitute anti-oppressive practice. It will provide an overview of the processes of empowerment, advocacy, service user and carer participation and promoting citizenship.

Empowerment

Empowerment and advocacy are related concepts and strategies. In this portfolio approach to anti-oppressive practice we will examine the different aspects of each approach. Adams' definition of empowerment is a useful starting point:

> the capacity of individuals, groups and/or communities to take control of their circumstances, exercise power and achieve their own goals, and the process by which, individually and collectively, they are able to help themselves and others to maximize the quality of their lives.
>
> (Adams 2008: 7)

Mackay (2007) argues that there are three main theoretical strands (which are not mutually exclusive), to empowerment which are summarised below:

- *Exit*: 'Voting with your feet', which is associated with the consumer movement, with regard to changing products if dissatisfied. He notes that in social work '[t]his idea seems realistic where service users have control or influence over a budget' (Mackay 2007: 270) and cites direct payments as a current example of this.

- *Voice*: 'Having a say', which is about 'attempting to influence and change and improve services' (2007: 270). He suggests that this does exist in social services, for example in service user and carer participation in committees, consultations, etc. The issue here is ensuring that when views and opinions are voiced social workers and social services actively listen to them, and take them into account when making decisions.

- *Rights*: 'Power to exercise rights which we all have', which are based on legislation and citizenship (Mackay 2007: 270). This approach necessitates that service users are aware of their rights and of how to pursue them.

So, what is the role of the social worker in empowering service users and what processes can be used in practice to ensure effective empowerment. Empowerment can take place at a number of levels. Adams (2008) provides a framework of how to aid practitioners in empowering individuals, groups, organisations, and communities and political systems. Empowering approaches in working with individuals requires using skills to overcome disabling barriers, such as working with someone to build their self-confidence, accessing relevant knowledge and developing thinking and action skills. The core skills of communication, assessment and planning are necessary components to empowering individuals. It is important to avoid a simplistic approach to empowerment, which merely emphasises that the service user 'should do things for themselves'. Modelling is a useful technique as it can provide the service user with practical examples of how to undertake tasks such as approaching organisations for assistance, or confronting individuals or organisations. Coaching is a related technique and involves the social worker working alongside a service user, supporting and advising. However, Trevithick (2005) warns against a mechanistic use of tools and techniques, and reinforces the importance of relationships, developing a mutual understanding of issues, and working together to build capacity in individuals.

Adams (2008: 173) provides a synopsis of the stages of group empowerment as provided in four different texts. The framework he provides is summarised from Lee (2001: 308–50) and gives a useful starting point for considering the elements in empowering groups.

Beginning phase of work:

1. meeting and taking stock of the group;

2. formation of the group;

3. defining empowerment goals together;

4. choosing a theme to begin with.

The work phase:

5. using social work skills to develop the mutual aid power of the group;

6. members encouraged by social worker to pose challenging questions;

7. group members asked to share feelings and analyse on personal, institutional and system levels;

8. group develops tools for raising consciousness;

9. as the tools are questioned, the group consciousness becomes more critical;

10. group develops options for action: personally, institutionally and politically;

11. group members take action;

12. group reflection on action continues until members decide the action is complete.

Mackay (2007) and Adams (2008) liken empowerment strategies to advocacy – a concept and process which is further explored below.

Advocacy

Advocacy movements have developed over the last twenty years, initially in the fields of learning disability, disability and mental health. Donnison proposes that '[t]here is no single thing that the term advocacy describes' (Donnison 2009: 21). His text provides a wide-ranging discussion of advocacy with practice examples in the areas of what advocates do in different individual, group and community settings. He suggests that there are eight main kinds of advocacy (with regard to advocacy for people with mental health difficulties or learning disabilities where advocacy is most strong). These are:

1. informal or natural advocates – these people would have no formal qualifications;

2. political advocacy – by elected representatives at all levels of government;

3. advocacy by professionals for their own patients or clients;

4. self-advocacy – people speak up for themselves with varying amounts of support;

5. peer advocacy – people who are supported by people with similar experiences to themselves;

6. parents' and carers' advocacy for the people they are looking after;

7. citizens' advocacy in which an individual volunteer gives support to one person – their 'partner';

8. professional advocacy – conducted by professionally trained advocates for their client.

(adapted from Donnison 2009: 21–2)

In his text he also introduces the concept of 'issue-based advocacy' (Donnison 2009: 23) which are movements that establish themselves in response to particular issues.

There is an ongoing debate in social work literature about the efficacy of the use of advocates. On the one hand advocacy is viewed as having an important role in the overall movement to identify the causes of unnecessary suffering as external to the individual. On the other hand, some writers suggest that professional advocates may unintentionally compound powerlessness and stigma in their representation of people (Adams 2009).

As social work students you will most likely be involved in undertaking advocacy as a professional, that is advocating for service users, but not as a professionally trained advocate such as a lawyer. In doing so you may be making use of the advocacy skills which fit within the generic social work skills that you develop. However, while you may represent the views of a service user to your own, or another organisation, and lobby on their behalf, it is unlikely that you will be able to work with the autonomy of an independent advocate. Mackay (2007) acknowledges the conflict of interest that social workers may find when faced with the requirement to undertake legal and professional duties and, at the same time, uphold the needs and rights of the service user. He suggests certain core principles of empowerment and advocacy including:

- building and sustaining a culture of listening;

- safeguarding legal rights;

- acknowledging the power of social workers;

- being authentic and having congruent professional traits and values;

- acknowledging responsibility of the culture of organisations;

- developing skills to challenge ethical dilemmas;

- having principles of no harm;

- reflecting in an enquiring and humble manner.

(adapted from Mackay 2007: 282)

A further issue to consider is that you may be working with service users who are part of a self-advocacy group, have the support of a citizen advocate or have an independent advocate who is their representative in dealings with social service or health organisations. So, as a representative of your organisation, you will be responding directly to the advocate of the service user. Your professional views as a social worker may well differ from those of the service user. Typically, this conflict arises where there are different assessments of the level of risk involved in any particular situation. The complexities of service user involvement are further discussed below.

Service user and carer participation and involvement

A parallel and related development alongside the growth of advocacy in social services has been the growth of service user and carer involvement in the planning and delivery of both social work services and social work education. The term *service user and carer* is a well-recognised one. It refers to people who use or may potentially make use of social work services either on their own behalf or on behalf of others, for whom they are caring. However, the term is not without its critics. At a fundamental level, concern has been expressed that the term 'user' has unfortunate pejorative connotations. At a more political level, the term is considered by some to reduce a person's identity to that of a user of services, with possible implications of passivity. This is a service provider's view of the relationship. The Shaping Our Lives Network (2003) has argued that service users should always self-identify as service users and should not be labelled as such. Some concern has been expressed in carers' organisations that the coupling of the two terms service user and carer does not sufficiently distinguish between the two groups who may have very different needs and agendas. However, a further complication that arises in defining a person in receipt of services is that a person may be using such services both in the role of a service user and as a carer. An older person may need assistance with some aspects of personal care, but also be the main carer for a partner. A person in receipt of assistance for substance misuse issues might also be the carer of a disabled child. A person providing care for a disabled partner may also be subject to domestic abuse by that partner. These issues relate to the discussion of the complexities of identity discussed in the previous chapter. Finally, in respect of terminology, other terms have been used, for example service experts, experts by expertise or service participants, but as service user and carer is the most common term used in social work, this term will be used in this text, although with an acknowledgement of the inadequacies of the term.

Braye (2000) has identified three kinds of mandates which have influenced the development of service user and carer participation in social work provision: legal and policy, professional and service user. In legal and policy mandates the rights of service users and carers have been highlighted in successive laws and policy guidance over the last twenty years. Examples of this are child care legislation, in which the views and rights of children are highlighted (The Children Act, 1989; The Children (Scotland) Act, 1995), and legislation which has introduced direct payments for disabled people (The Community Care Direct Payment Act, 1996). Two professional mandates are identified by Braye (2000). One is based on professional codes of practice which stipulate that adherence should be paid to the rights and choices of users of services. The second is based on a professional value base which seeks to promote equal opportunities and respect diversities. The final mandate comes from service user organisations themselves, developing from movements such as the disability movement discussed in the previous chapter.

There are a range of ways in which service users and carers participate in social work provision. These have been identified by Smith as *strategies* on a continuum of participation and involvement: compliance; non-cooperation; resistance; challenge; collaboration and control (2008: 125–41).

At the least empowering end of the continuum, service users and carers' relationship with social services is characterised by *compliance*. In these situations service users choose or are required to comply with the requirements of the organisation. This may be because they feel that lack of compliance could result in a service being withdrawn. For instance, a parent in receipt of child care provision may not agree with a social worker's assessment of their parenting skills but is in need of the child care service in order to undertake training or employment. Another major reason for compliance is that the service user is legally obliged to cooperate with the service or may risk more intensive intervention or loss of liberty by not doing so. Examples of such compliance may be: where parents have been subject to initial child protection inquiries and a family assessment is taking place; where a young person is subject to a supervision or monitoring order in the community as an alternative to a custodial sentence; or where a person with mental health problems is being supervised in the community following discharge from hospital.

Non-cooperation is the second strategy identified by Smith (2008). He suggests that this may be straightforward, and cites an example of a service user deciding not to turn up for drug treatment and testing. In instances of child protection, parents may not cooperate because they are concerned about social work assessment and observation of their parenting. In the case of Victoria Climbié (Laming 2003), examples were seen of parental non-cooperation and also feigned compliance. However, there may be other elements to non-cooperation. For example, failure of service users to turn up to appointments may not be due to their resistance to assistance but due to lack of understanding of the social work process, or failure to be kept informed of such process or as a result of lack of personal resources. Smith (2008) argues that rather than seeing non-cooperation always in a negative light, it should also be considered as a legitimate response to the frequent lack of communication between services and service users, and to service users' feelings of being estranged from the social work process.

Smith (2008) suggests that resistance is the first of the more purposeful strategies adopted by service users and that it differs from non-cooperation as it is more intentional. In resisting, service users begin to take part in agenda setting. So a parent who chooses a resistant strategy to the relationship with social services would adopt a different approach to that taken by the parent given as an example in the discussion on compliance. They could use ways to lobby the social work department through written communication or attendance at meetings. Smith cautions that it is important not to romanticise resistant behaviour by service users as 'it may not always lead to desirable outcomes' (Smith 2008: 136). For example there may be legitimate professional concerns in the child protection situation posed above and a change of assessment might not be in the best interest of the child or parent. Smith suggests this service user strategy requires social workers to develop skills in renegotiating engagement and intervention.

Challenge as a strategy is one which Smith (2008) argues is influenced by a rights-led agenda, and is likely to be a more confrontational approach in which the authority of the service provider is challenged. In this approach the service user may use formal procedures such as complaints procedures and legal interventions.

Collaboration could be seen as a less active strategy than challenge, however, Smith (2008) argues that active engagement, participation and involvement of service users in service provision, even where the service user may disagree with the position of the service provider, can result in productive and meaningful partnerships and good outcomes. He cites family group conferences, in which a range of family members and friends and professionals meet in a collaborative way to share information and agree ways forward, with the discussion being led by members of the family (Family Rights Group n.d.).

Finally, a control strategy is where service users would 'seek complete control over the way in which needs are defined, rights are exercised and interventions are determined' (Smith 2008: 141). This type of strategy would not be effective in many statutory settings where legal duties and powers would mean the control of the service by service users would not be possible or desirable. However, examples of this have been seen in self-management services such as Centres for Integrated Living (Oliver 1990) and, on an individual level, the introduction of direct payments. The Community Care (Direct Payments) Act, 1996 has been seen as an example of the move towards user control of services (Smith 2008).

A comprehensive summary of barriers to service user and carer participation and benefits of participation, with reference to research is given by Warren (2007), and is summarised below.

Potential barriers to participation:

- lack of awareness by people that they have a right to participate;

- social invisibility of some people, for example, those who do not want to identify as having an illness;

- lack of self-esteem and support;

- lack of dedicated funding and resources;

- lack of accessible information;

- stereotyping of service users by providers.

(adapted from Warren 2007: 21)

Potential benefits of participation:

- influences provision directly;

- increases confidence and self-esteem;

- develops self help and mutual support;

- provides a personal therapeutic experience;

- empowers through collective involvement;

- provides opportunities for learning;

- provides new role models;
- develops peer-led initiatives.

(adapted from Warren 2007: 25–6)

However, in spite of the benefits identified above, Cowden and Singh (2007) caution against taking an uncritical view of service user involvement. They express concern that some service users have become professional experts or consultants, servicing the needs of service providers rather than those of service users and carers. They argue for 'critical dialogue' (Cowden and Singh 2007: 5) between service users and professionals.

Promoting citizenship

While the citizenship agenda has been part of service user and carer movements since the early 1990s, Dalrymple and Burke (2006) identify that it has been a political concept since the start of the welfare state in the UK, and the concept was revisited by UK governments in the 1990s. They advise that citizenship is a concept which has been used by both the right and left of the political spectrum. Viewed positively it 'implies empowerment, membership and rights' (Dalrymple and Burke 2006: 148) but it has also been used to exclude members of society. Dalrymple and Burke (2006) cite immigration processes as an example of this. The active involvement of service users in developing a range of services is a positive step towards promoting citizenship.

It might appear to you that this level of involvement is beyond your capacity or role; however, smaller incremental steps to promoting citizenship are feasible.

In the final section of this chapter, based on the concepts and processes discussed in these two chapters on understanding anti-oppressive theory and practice, we will draw together the key areas for consideration in a practice situation.

Putting anti-oppressive theories and processes into practice situations: the 'ARARAE' framework

Awareness

Awareness of the forms and processes of oppression is an early stage in developing anti-oppressive practice. This requires research into the particular practice situation that you are presented with either in practice learning or in the form of a case study. The major social divisions identified in the previous chapter are a starting point. There is substantial research evidence with regard to social inequalities and marginalisation of certain social groups. However, given that individual and social identities are complex, awareness of the particular potential for inequality and oppression in each individual situation is required.

Recognition

A theoretical awareness of potential forms of inequality, marginalisation and oppression does not necessarily mean that these processes are recognised in any given situation. In practice, you need to be able to use academic learning to assist recognition of aspects of oppression, which may often be hidden. What approaches to social divisions outlined in the last chapter might be particularly pertinent to this situation?

Analysis

Building on an awareness of the processes of oppression, an analysis of the situation is required. Consider the implications of the power relationship between yourself and the service user. What questions do you need to consider with regard to issues of identities and cultures?

Reflection

Following an analysis of the processes of oppression, it is useful to hypothesise about the situation, that is, to consider the different possible interpretations as to processes of oppression, considering who is involved and what the different relational power operations may be.

Action planning

Having reflected on the analysis and having developed one or more hypotheses, a plan of action can be drawn up. With regard to a case study in an academic assignment, this might mean the planning of how you will address issues of oppression when writing your assignment. In a practice learning setting, this might mean preparing a plan of action for your supervision session with your practice teacher.

Evaluation

This involves periodic evaluation of your work. Reflection is an important aspect of evaluation; however, evaluation is a more systematic process in which you reflect on the process of intervention so far. Here you would return to your original analysis and action planning and review your work. How would you involve the service user in this situation?

Exercise 1

Sana is a lone parent with three children, aged three, five and nine. She moved to the UK from Iraq four years previously. Since coming to the UK she has separated from her husband. Her first language is Arabic. She can read and write in English. She has no extended family. She and her children live in small rented accommodation which is poorly maintained. Sana has contacted social services on a number of previous occasions for assistance with financial issues, housing and child care issues. Her two older children attend the local school. Her youngest child is considered to have developmental delays but there is no diagnosis and the child is being monitored by health services.

She comes to the social services department with similar issues as on previous occasions: financial, housing and child care issues. The child care issues on this occasion involve her ongoing concern with regard to her youngest child's development. While her health visitor makes regular monitoring visits Sana states that she has had no information from the GP or hospital consultant about a diagnosis or future plans. Her housing issues relate to the lack of repairs being undertaken in the flat. Of particular concern are poorly fitting windows which cannot be closed and a shower unit which is in need of repair. The flat is damp and expensive to heat.

At the time Sana comes to the office she does not have an allocated social worker. You have seen her previously on two occasions and have assisted with financial issues in the past. Although Sana has come to the office she states: 'I've come to see what you can do. I don't know why I've come because it made no difference last time. Things are still just as bad. The landlord still doesn't take any notice when I tell him and the hospital still haven't got back.'

Using the 'ARARAE' framework, identify how you might begin to analyse Sana's situation and begin to prepare to work in an anti-oppressive way.

Exercise 2

Michael is a black male, aged twenty-five, who lives at home with his parents in a local authority flat. He has a learning disability. He attends a centre during the day and has indicated to staff that he wants to leave home and live with another female member of the day centre.

- Consider the power relations in which Michael finds himself.

- What multiple identities might Michael have?

- How would you plan to work with Michael in an empowering way?

- Explicitly identify the principles you would intend to use.

- What particular skills do you need to develop to work with Michael?

Key learning points

- A number of inter-related theoretical strands underpin the concept of empowerment.

- There is a debate with regard to whether statutory social workers can be advocates, but they can use advocacy skills.

- Service user and carer participation takes a variety of forms. The kind of form is likely to be influenced by the basis on which the relationship between social worker and service user is formed.

Further reading

Adams, R. (2008) *Empowerment, participation and social work*, Basingstoke: Palgrave Macmillan.

Dalrymple, J. and Burke, B. (2006) *Anti-oppressive practice*, Maidenhead: McGraw-Hill.

7 Assessment

In this chapter the principles of assessment will be considered. Definitions will be provided, a range of assessments will be described and theoretical approaches to assessment will be summarised. An overview will be given of the assessment process and illustrations will be given of specific assessment tools. You will be directed to appropriate social work literature on assessment. The chapter will end by showing how different textbooks approach the discussion of assessment and will provide students with a framework to help them decide on which approaches assist their understanding of assessment.

The ability to assess is a core skill of social work practice, and there is much material in the literature on social work theory and practice. However as Crisp *et al.* note, 'a common understanding may not be apparent to the novice reader' (2005: 16). Elsewhere, they also argue that '[a]lthough assessment has been recognised as a core skill in social work and should underpin social work interventions, there is no singular theory or understanding as to what the purpose of assessment is and what the process should entail' (Crisp *et al.* 2003: 5).

Definitions

Assessment is not a single event, it is an ongoing process, in which the client participates or service user participates, the purpose of which is to assist the social worker to understand people in relation to their environment. Assessment is also . . . a basis for planning what needs to be done to maintain, improve or bring about change in the person, the environment or both.

(Coulshed and Orme 2006: 24)

Assessment is the foundation for all effective interventions; as such it needs to be grounded in evidence from research and theory in disciplines such as sociology and psychology, which illuminate human need.

(Baldwin and Walker 2009: 209)

assessment is both an art and a science since it involves wisdom, skills, appreciation of diversity and systematically applied knowledge in practice.

(Parker and Bradley 2007: 4)

It can be seen that there are common elements to these definitions but also different emphases. Therefore, it is important to read a range of texts on assessment to ascertain the variety of approaches and to consider which approaches best fit the needs of the service user, your value base, and the social work context in order that you can appropriately integrate theory and practice.

Range of assessments

While the above definitions emphasise that assessment is a process, the nature of an assessment can vary considerably with regard to legislative context, purpose of assessment (for example, focus on need or risk), ownership of the assessment, time frame in which the assessment has to be completed, and the multi-disciplinary nature of assessments.

Legislative and policy context

Consideration needs to be given to the legislative context and the particular requirements of the law with regard to the content and process of assessment. In the four countries that make up the UK there are different legislative requirements and, following from this, different policy frameworks for social workers in the fields of child care, community care and, in Scotland, criminal justice. So, with regard to preparation, a careful reading of the legislative and policy context is required and students should ensure that they refer to the literature which discusses their own country's framework as there are some subtle but important differences between the countries. This does not mean that literature which discusses legislation and policy in one country is not a useful source to help critique policy in another country. Indeed, comparisons are useful ways to develop critical analyses; however, students need to be explicit about the origin of the legislation.

Purpose of assessment

Assessments may be required for a variety of purposes and may be undertaken with individuals, groups or communities. Assessments may be required by legislation and governmental policy frameworks. Social workers may be required to produce reports for courts, children's panels (Scotland) and tribunals, and to adhere to statutory guidance. Assessments, such as the range of assessments in community and adult care, may be required by statute but not presented to bodies such as courts but rather to resource panels, which may be single or multi-agency. These kinds of assessments which produce formal reports will usually be required to be completed within a fixed time scale to meet statutory deadlines. On production of the report the worker completing it may have no more involvement with the service user after decisions are made with regard to risk or need.

Exercise 1

Assessment: No further service

Justyna is a twenty-year-old white young woman, living in Scotland, who was found guilty of shoplifting. The court requested that the Social Work Department provide a report on her background. The social worker undertakes an assessment, gathering information on Justyna's background and attitude to her offence. The report was completed with a recommendation that probation would not be a suitable disposal and that a fine be considered. The fine was the disposal.

Although the production of an assessment report in itself is a process, it might also be a 'one-off' event in the sense of the involvement of a particular social worker, but the service user may receive services from another part of the agency or a related agency. If the assessment results in the service user receiving services from another social worker in another agency, then the assessment process will begin again, but in a different form.

Exercise 2

Assessment: Transfer to another team

David is a white seventy-two-year-old man living with his wife. He has been in hospital for a hip replacement. The social worker based in the hospital has assessed David's needs on discharge. A community care assessment has been made and a plan has been constructed by

---

the hospital social worker. On discharge a community-based social work agency is contacted and David is allocated a worker from this team. The worker receives the community care plan which forms the basis of the involvement. However, the worker also undertakes a new assessment as David's circumstances begin to change.

On the other hand, an assessment may take place over a longer period of time, may be undertaken by workers in statutory or voluntary agencies, but be less formal in nature.

Exercise 3

Assessment: Longer term

Joseph is a nineteen-year-old black man who lives alone. He has been referred to the social worker by his general practitioner, who has prescribed antidepressants but who considers that he needs a range of social supports. Joseph left residential care two years ago. A social worker is allocated to Joseph and begins an assessment of his needs and strengths in order to work with him to improve his situation. There is no time limit on this assessment and no formal report is produced. The process and outcome of the assessment is recorded in case notes and discussed in supervision.

Needs assessment

The term 'needs assessment' is usually taken to refer to assessment in the field of community care, as in Example 2 above. The emphasis in needs assessment is that the focus is on the specific and diverse needs of the service user and carer. From the assessment follows a plan or care package, the aim of which is to bring together resources from a range of agencies. A needs assessment aims to start with the service user's situation, and not with an assessment of the eligibility of the person to receive resources an agency can provide. In the above examples, the needs of the service user will be a focus of attention alongside other considerations such as risk to others and risk to self.

Risk assessment

In all the examples given above there is an element of the assessment of risk. In the last decade there has been an increasing concern with the assessment of risk, and a range of risk assessment tools, which workers are required to use, have been produced at national and agency level. The broad principles of risk assessment are that a thorough examination needs to take place of: a person assessed as a poser of risk; a person assessed as being at risk; behaviour which is seen as being risky; how to accurately identify risk; and the extent to which the risk is acceptable (Kemshall 2002). Concern has been expressed that a simplistic attitude to risk assessment has emerged. This attitude is based on the premise that it is possible to eliminate all risks and does not acknowledge that social workers are required to practise in conditions of uncertainty (Parton 1998). Risk is socially constructed and how risky a situation is seen to be depends upon the social and legal context and the perceptions and understandings of those involved. Over-concentration on risk can lead to defensive and risk-averse practice – that is, where social workers are disinclined to take any risk and the rights of the service user may be compromised (Barry 2007). There is growing attention to the process of risk management, where the aim is to identify risk factors and to work to remove or reduce them by strengthening protective factors and supports, and improving coping strategies (Kemshall 2002; Barry 2007).

Multi-disciplinary assessments

Increasingly, assessments are jointly undertaken by a range of professionals who may use a common or single assessment framework. Each worker assesses the situation from their skill and knowledge base and contributes to the final assessment.

Exercise 4

Assessment: Multi-disciplinary

Peter and Mary are both in their seventies. They both have restricted mobility and between them have a range of health and social care needs. A multi-disciplinary assessment is undertaken with inputs from social work, community-based health professionals such as the general practitioner, district nurse, and the community psychiatric nurse, and a hospital-based consultant.

Summary of key features of theories of assessment

The literature on assessment in social work varies considerably in how explicitly it explains the theoretical, evidence and value base of assessment. Smale *et al.*'s (1993) work is much quoted in the literature on assessment. These authors proposed three models of assessment: the questioning model, the procedural model and the exchange model.

The questioning model

In this model the workers identify the information to be gathered, gather this from service users and other key informants, determine the problem, and recommend solutions. The social worker is seen as the professional expert who determines and provides solutions to a problem. This model has been criticised as one in which the social worker has a pre-determined theoretical basis for conducting the assessment, and is mainly used when the focus of the assessment is on risk (Milner and O'Byrne 2009). On the other hand, it has been argued that a systematic approach to questioning in which information, views and perspectives are sought on a variety of areas and from a range of sources can be empowering (Coulshed and Orme 2006).

The procedural model

A worker adopting a procedural model to assessment would be likely to use a fixed agency tool or framework. The emphasis here tends to be also on assessing risk, ascertaining eligibility for a service and allocating resources; it has been criticised as encouraging a 'one-way process' (Coulshed and Orme 2006: 31).

The exchange model

Smale *et al.* (1993) argue that service users are the experts on their own experiences and that the process of assessment is one undertaken jointly by the service user or carer and the social worker. The role of the social worker is to assist the service user to articulate their needs and possible solutions and to create a support network working alongside the social worker.

Narrative approaches

Fook proposes an alternative to the above models. She argues that 'a new approach ... involves a broad recognition that the act of assessing involves creating a set of meanings which function discursively' (Fook 2002: 118). Fook suggests that traditional approaches to assessment are based on assumptions that assessment is a linear process, that professionals maintain the power and that they are undertaken with preconceived ideas about underlying causes and solutions. She maintains that assessments need to allow for multiple understandings of a situation. Workers need to understand that, in making an assessment, they are producing their own professional *narrative* or story about what is going on and why. This narrative is required to be constructed by continually checking assumptions and by being mindful that the aim is that it works in favour of the service user. In doing so, the power of the professional is acknowledged, as is the fact that professional judgement needs to be made. However, this judgement is arrived at after ongoing critical reflection of a range of perspectives.

The assessment process: overview

The process of assessment is variously described in the literature. A search of the literature provides a range of approaches. Texts can be more or less detailed about the content and process of assessment. Some texts provide examples of questions that could be used in the assessment process, for example Hepworth *et al.* (2002) provide an example of an interview guide. Some, often examining assessment in relation to work with specific service user groups, provide information on specific assessment frameworks, for example in the field of sexual abuse assessments (Calder 2009). Others offer an over-view of the assessment process, for example:

1. *Preparing* for the task;

2. *Collecting data* including perceptions of the service user; the family and other agencies of the problems and any attempted solutions;

3. *Applying professional knowledge* (practice wisdom as well as theory) to seek analysis, under-standing or interpretation of data;

4. *Making judgements* about the relationships, needs, risks, standard of care or safety, seriousness of the situation, and people's capacities and potential for coping or for change (is the progress good enough?);

5. *Deciding and/or recommending what is to be done*, plus how, by whom and when and how progress will be evaluated.

(Milner and O'Byrne 2009: 4)

Milner and O'Byrne (2009) develop this summary with a helpful suggestion of what needs to be considered at each stage of the assessment process, so for example with regard to *preparation* for assessment they suggest:

- Make a list of key informants – people, documents, agencies. Keep this on file so that gaps in the information source are clearly visible.

- Prepare a schedule for collecting data from *all* key informants. Adapt agency checklists for this purpose.

- Decide on an interview schedule. If it is inappropriate to use an open interview format, make a list of essential questions to which answers are needed. Keep this on file, but give copies to the informants where this would be helpful.

- Prepare a statement of intent that includes purpose, what one is able to do, limits, and how one will be accountable for one's values. Although this may be given orally to potential service users, keep a copy on file.

- Make a note of early (tentative) explanations.

(Milner and O'Byrne 2009: 61)

Milner and O'Byrne's (2009) overview can be usefully used in a range of assessments as it offers a flexible approach to the assessment process.

The assessment process: tools and frameworks

While undertaking an assessment guided by the broad process such as that provided by Milner and O'Byrne (2009), social workers may, or may be required to, make use of specific assessment frameworks and tools.

Frameworks

Crisp *et al.* (2005) evaluate a range of assessment frameworks used by social workers. They argue that assessment frameworks, which have explicit theoretical or conceptual underpinnings and are built around a validated evidence base, can offer workers systematic professional guidance. Assessment frameworks may assist workers to be more explicit about the evidence base for their recommendations, be that information gathered in practice or research evidence. However, by providing fixed 'domain' frameworks, they may encourage workers to seek only evidence that is requested in the framework (a tick-box approach) and not to search for different kinds of evidence and understandings. In their analysis of four assessment frameworks Crisp *et al.* (2005) found that:

- There was no agreement about what constitutes an assessment framework.

- Assessment frameworks vary considerably in the amount of detail and topics covered.

- Different assumptions are made about the reader's knowledge base.

- A key purpose in all frameworks was the assessment or risk.

- There is little discussion of the theoretical underpinnings of the assessment process.

- There is some discussion of the use of research evidence to underpin assessment.

- There are expectations that assessments are grounded in evidence.

- Some assessment frameworks include specific structured tools.

- It is commonly accepted that assessments are multi-disciplinary.

- Partnership with service users is a core principle.

(Adapted from Crisp *et al.* 2005: 61)

Specific tools

Parker and Bradley (2007) provide a useful summary of assessment tools which can be used in the assessment process, which are summarised below.

Genogram   A family tree which shows family relationships in a diagrammatic way. It shows how close or distanced family members are and can show current and historical relationships. Completing the genogram can assist both service users and workers to understand the development of relationships and current issues in the family.

Ecomap   A map of the person or family in the social environment. It identifies family and wider social networks, community resources and involvement of a range of agencies with which the family have contact.

Culturagram   This combines elements of the genogram and the ecomap but focuses on the impact and meaning of different aspects of family and social culture on the family's situation.

Flow diagram and life road map   These tools can provide a chronology of the life of an individual or family. Changes over time can be charted and significant events noted and discussed.

(Parker and Bradley 2007)

Reading the textbooks on assessment

The previous sections have summarised the literature on assessment available in social work literature. In this final section we will use the work of Crisp *et al.* (2005) to consider how you can begin to analyse the content of textbooks on assessment. A framework for analysis is provided to help you decide on which approaches assist your understanding of assessment.

In their analysis of those textbooks which include a substantial discussion of assessment, Crisp *et al.* (2005) note the different focuses of assessment in different texts. They found that attention to assessment in the texts they reviewed varied from 2 to 45 per cent. Texts varied in how explicit they were with regard to the theoretical base of assessment. There was also considerable difference in the extent to which the authors made specific reference to the evidence base or research evidence which informed their discussion. For example, they found that Milner and O'Byrne (2002), Clifford (1998) and Parker and Bradley (2003) all discuss how adequate the research evidence is with regard to their suggested approaches to assessment. Similarly, although the importance of the legislative context was acknowledged by many authors, the amount of detail given about the legislative basis of assessment varied across textbooks. It is important to note that the lack of inclusion of such details is not necessarily a criticism, given that legislation can change very quickly. Textbooks varied considerably in the amount of attention given to service users' and carer users' participation in assessment and their perspective on the process, and very few texts had separate chapters on anti-oppressive practice. Textbooks on assessment also vary in terms of their target audience, so you will need to ensure that the textbook is aimed at social work students and to consider the usefulness of the text for your stage of academic and practice learning.

Crisp *et al.* (2005) provide two frameworks to assist the reader in identifying the differences of focus and content in textbooks on assessment and in assessment frameworks, and suggest these are used in assessing their relevance and value. Table 7.1 is an adaptation of Crisp *et al.*'s (2005) frameworks, designed specifically to assist you in evaluating the textbooks on assessment that you are reading.

Table 7.1
Guidance for evaluation of textbooks on social work assessment

Definitions	Do the authors define assessment; if so, how? Did they provide a new definition? Did they refer to definitions provided by previous authors? If so, are these definitions critiqued?
Theoretical underpinnings	Do the authors explicitly mention theoretical underpinnings of assessment? If so what underpinnings do they identify? Are they critiqued? Do the authors propose a new theoretical approach towards assessment?
Evidence / research base	What evidence base for assessment is referred to in the text?
Legislation / legal frameworks	Is reference made to legislation?
Process of assessment	Is the process of assessment discussed and analysed? What specific frameworks or tools are discussed and analysed?
Information obtained during the assessment process	Does the text identify the kinds of information needed in an assessment? If so, what kinds of information are suggested? Are suggestions made about the way information is gathered? What discussion is there of the analysis of the information?
Needs assessment	Is a definition of need given? If so, how is it defined? What suggestions are given to assist the identification of need?
Risk assessment	Is a definition of risk given? If so, how is it defined? Is the assessment of risk critically analysed?
Multi-disciplinary assessment	What attention is given to multi-disciplinary assessments?
Involvement of service users and carers in the process	What attention is given to the involvement of users and carers in the assessment process? Is any feedback provided on service users' and carers' views of the assessment process?
Language other than English and the use of interpreters	Does the text discuss how the needs of service users and carers who use a language other than spoken English are addressed?

Source: Adapted from Crisp *et al.* 2005

In this chapter an overview of definitions and processes of assessment has been given. Students have been directed to core texts in this field. A framework and guidance for the analysis of textbooks has been provided. To conclude, it is important to acknowledge the limitations of an analysis of literature only. In order to integrate theory into practice, students need to use the analysis to inform their assessment practice. As Crisp *et al.* (2005) note:

> Readers should not assume that they will develop expertise in assessment only by reading relevant textbooks and assessment frameworks. Attempting learning exercises contained in textbooks and assessment frameworks, discussion of concepts and practices in supervision, and ultimately attempting to put the theory into practice, are all further steps in becoming a skilled practitioner.
>
> (Crisp *et al.* 2005: 67)

Exercise 1

Choose one chapter on assessment from a social work textbook and evaluate it using the above framework and guidance. Then summarise:

- What are the most useful aspects of the text?

- What aspects are missing from this text?

- Where would you now look to seek out information on the missing aspects?

Exercise 2

In your own words, building on the literature summarised in this chapter write three short paragraphs:

- a broad definition of assessment;

- a definition of needs assessment; and

- a definition of risk assessment.

What do you not feel sure about and how will you find this out?

Key learning points

- There is no singular understanding of the purposes or processes of assessment.

- There is a range of assessment frameworks, but all are primarily concerned with assessing needs and/or risks.

- Social work texts offer different material on assessment, so it is important to find out their strengths and weaknesses, and use a range of social work literature.

Further reading

Milner, J. and O'Byrne, P. (2009) *Assessment in social work*, 3rd edn, Basingstoke: Palgrave Macmillan.

Parker, J. and Bradley, G. (2007) *Social work practice*, Exeter: Learning Matters.

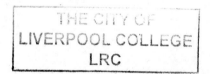

8 Beginning to understand social work methods

The chapter will provide an overview of the range of social work methods of intervention and then will focus on two methods of intervention – psychosocial work and task-centred work – using three core social work textbooks written by Coulshed and Orme (2006), Milner and O'Byrne (2009) and Payne (2005). A preliminary summary of the origins, theoretical underpinnings and core principles, processes and techniques of, and critical commentaries on, the two methods will be presented, based on the material provided in these three textbooks. The final section of the chapter will examine how the process of understanding can be deepened by suggesting how you can further your learning and deepen your understanding drawing on Stage 3: Systematic Data Collection provided in Chapter 4.

In their critiques, the three key authors cited above carefully acknowledge and reference the authors whose ideas they summarise and adapt. Although at the first stages of learning about social work method, students may use bullet-point summaries as shown below, in order to develop an overview of each method, it is important that students take the same care as the authors in ensuring they acknowledge their original sources and when they are using secondary texts, using the referencing system required by their university.

Definitions

In the social work literature a variety of terms are used to describe methods of social work intervention. Payne offers the following definitions:

> A theory is an organised statement of ideas about the world. . . . In social work, the term theory covers three different possibilities:
>
> *Models* describe what happens during practice in a general way, in a wide range of situations, and in a structured form, so that they can extract certain principles and patterns of activity which give practice consistency. Models help you to structure and organise how you approach a complicated situation. A good example is task centred practice . . .
>
> *Perspectives* express values or views of the world which allow participants to order their minds sufficiently to be able to manage themselves while participating. Perspectives help you think about what is happening in an organised way. Applying different perspectives can help you see situations from different points of view. Examples of perspectives are feminist . . . or systems theories . . .
>
> *Explanatory theory* accounts for why an action results and causes particular consequences and identifies the circumstances in which it does so. Some writers reserve the word 'theory' to ideas that offer causal explanation. To them theories have to tell you 'what works'. Cognitive behavioural theory . . . is an example of explanatory theory.
>
> (Payne 2005: 5)

Payne explains that the focus of his book is theories of '*how to do social work*', that is, practice theories (2005: 7). Coulshed and Orme differentiate between 'theories for practice' which constitute foundational knowledge such as psychology and sociology, 'theories of practice' such as task-centred practice and 'theories from practice . . . derived from someone's experience written down and shared with others' (2006: 12–15). Finally, in their 'aim to provide a way through the thicket of concepts and theories of which social workers become aware in seeking helpful explanations for the nature of people and society and to locate some signposts' (2009: 67), Milner and O'Byrne use the very useful analogy of choosing an appropriate map for social work intervention.

The range of methods of intervention

There are a range of methods of intervention in social work. The way in which the three core texts discussed in this chapter are structured provides some indication of the different approaches to categorising and discussing methods. For example, in the section on methods of intervention in Coulshed and Orme (2006), the chapter titles which deal specifically with social work methods of intervention are entitled: Counselling; Working with loss and change; Task-centred practice; and Cognitive behavioural work; followed by a section on different contexts, e.g. working with families and children, and working with adults. In Payne (2005), in the second section of his book entitled 'Reviewing social work theories', chapters are entitled: Psychodynamic perspectives; Crisis intervention and task-centred methods; Cognitive behavioural theories; and Systems and ecological approaches, but there are also chapters in such areas as social psychology and social constructionism, and humanism and existentialism. Meanwhile, in Milner and O'Byrne (2009) the fourth chapter introduces the concepts of maps of intervention. This is then followed by chapters entitled: A map of the ocean: Psychodynamic approaches; An Ordnance Survey map: Behavioural approaches; A handy tourist map: Task-centred approaches; A navigator's map: Solution-focused approaches; and A forecast map: Narrative approaches. These chapters are followed by chapters on assessment in children's and adult services. When the contents of other social work method texts on methods of interventions are added to these, it can be seen that students at the beginning of their social work education may be a little overwhelmed.

Psychosocial approaches

Origins, theoretical underpinnings and core principles

Psychosocial methods of social work intervention are built on the work of Freud (1937). One of the most important Freudian concepts is *psychic determinism*, that is, that early experiences in childhood have a significant impact on people's adult lives. Freud developed a *personality theory* in which he argued that people operate consciously, unconsciously and pre-consciously. He suggests that people's *psyche* (the spiritual, emotional and motivational aspects of the mind) is composed of the *ego* which mainly operates in the conscious mind, and the *id* and *superego* which operate in the subconscious.

The superego 'develops through a process of internalisation' whereby a child internalises the 'values, rules, prohibitions and wishes of the parent or authority figure' (Milner and O'Byrne 2009: 85). Importantly, the emotional context of the internalisation is deeply influential, so emotional messages of anger, disdain and disappointment are also internalised. Consequently, the superego in adults may be restrictive and governed by feelings of guilt and instructions on what *should* or *ought to be* done. This is thought to result in such mental states as anxiety and depression. Alternatively, a child may have internalised messages which has led them to develop a highly permissive superego as an adult. This would manifest in a person having psychopathic or sociopathic tendencies – a person who has no internal rules governing her/his behaviour.

The id is also developed through processes of internalising early childhood experiences, and is often referred to as the animal drive or the wild unruly child part of the subconscious, governed by the *pleasure principle*. It is linked to instinctive urges and is considered to have two main drives, the *libido*, which is sexual impulse, desire and attraction, and the *mortido*, which is the killing instinct (Milner and O'Byrne 2009).

Finally the ego, placed between the superego and the id, is considered to be the Adult, Me or I, governed by the reality principle 'which thinks, decides, plans and relates to the world of *reality*' (Milner and O'Byrne 2009: 85). The ego strives to ensure predictability and stability, balancing the drives from the superego and the id.

Central to the psychodynamic understanding of people is an appreciation of *defence mechanisms* which the ego employs, positively or negatively, to cope with both internal and external events. Defence mechanisms can range from repression of feeling, denial, avoidance, projecting feelings on to others, splitting (where contradictory ideas and feelings are dealt with by dividing them into different mental compartments), and rationalisation (where emotionally unacceptable reasons for our or others' behaviour are repressed in favour of more acceptable ones).

The 1930s to 1970s saw the growth of psychosocial social work in the areas of individual therapy, counselling approaches and some forms of family work. Psychotherapy, based strictly on Freudian principles, took place mainly in psychiatric settings. However, the underlying principles have influenced more 'layperson' methods such as psychosocial and counselling approaches. Payne argues that the 'main issue in ego psychology practice is whether to be ego-supportive or ego-modifying' (2005: 89). Ego-modifying work would examine the influence of past experiences on current experiences and feelings, while ego-supportive work concentrates on current issues, using educative approaches and working with the current environment. Payne (2005) suggests that usually counselling is ego-modifying and social work is ego-strengthening. However, psychosocial social work which focuses on or includes consideration of building a relationship between worker and service user, often combines both practices. Hollis (1964, 1970) is probably the most influential proponent of psychosocial social work.

The processes and techniques of psychosocial social work

Coulshed and Orme (2006) provide a useful summary of Hollis's work (Hollis 1964, 1970). They explain that in psychosocial work:

- *Problems* are intra-psychic, interpersonal or environmental – relating to basic needs, for example love and trust.

- *Goals* are to understand and change the person, situation or both.

- *The client's role* is 'almost passive' and the client is encouraged to talk about thoughts and feelings, to bring them into consciousness and to increase *insight* or self-understanding.

- *The worker's role* is to use the relationship to study, diagnose and treat the person-in-situation, by establishing the relationship, building on ego strength, helping the client reach self-understanding and settle internal conflicts.

- *Techniques:*

    - *Sustaining* techniques include offering support by: assisting ventilation; giving realistic reassurance; offering acceptance; providing logical discussion; modelling coping behaviour; giving information; offering advice and guidance and manipulating the environment.

    - *Modifying* techniques to increase insight include: reflective communication; confrontation and clarification techniques which involve the use of interpretation.

        (adapted from Coulshed and Orme 2006: 112–15)

Critical commentaries on psychosocial casework

The authors of the three key texts in social work theory and practice have identified the following benefits and concerns of psychodynamic approaches including psychosocial social work. Below are summaries of their key points.

Advantages and benefits:

- influenced social work's open listening style of work;

- encourages exploration of feelings and unconscious factors;

- focuses on important areas of childhood and has led to the importance of attachment theory – which is well supported by research.

    (Payne 2005: 79)

- can assist you to question the obvious presenting problem;

- encourages an imaginative open-mindedness;

- assists our knowledge of how personalities function;

- encourages us to be cautious in labelling behaviour as abnormal;

- emphasises listening, understanding, accepting.

    (Coulshed and Orme 2006: 117–18)

- a useful way of understanding what appears to be irrational behaviour;

- the concept of defence mechanisms can assist the assessment of people who find it difficult to express emotions;

- understanding the influence of past events can be useful in understanding current surface behaviour;

- insight can empower people in self-understanding;

- useful in long-term work, for example with cases of deep-seated neurosis;

- has informed a listening and accepting approach.

(Milner and O'Byrne 2009: 91–2)

Disadvantages and concerns:

- a scientific and originally biological way of understanding people which does not take account of the right to self-determination, this focus detracts from more interpretative understanding of human behaviour;

- based on a 'medical model' of understanding human development and behaviour which assumes 'client' sickness with professional expertise leading to a cure;

- the importance of 'insight' in this cure model may mean that intervention ends when the client has gained an understanding of their problem and may not move to further more and supportive practical action;

- a range of cultural issues: the client may be seen as the problem and the cultural, social and political context not taken into account; the model is based on white European cultural norms;

- talking therapy may not be appropriate for less orally articulate clients.

(Payne 2005: 93–5)

- social workers are not mini-psychoanalysts;

- the terminology used may be difficult to understand;

- the approach may be too time consuming;

- the approach may encourage a simplistic blaming of the past and may not address current social and political inequalities;

- psychosocial casework has the oppressive potential to pathologise black clients, women, gay, lesbian and bisexual people;

- the approach is based on white middle-class norms with regard to self-awareness;

- there may be practitioners who operate a rigid, authoritarian practice which does not take into account difference, diversity and social and linguistic contexts.

(Coulshed and Orme 2006: 115–17)

- less successful in developing ways of working which are effective in terms of their cost or being accessible for service users;

- a number of writers have found that therapeutic interventions are not useful with certain service users, for example in instances of violence, child protection, or social problems;

- in Western culture the concept of emotion being better in than out has become common currency, but uncovering and showing feelings in some instances may be unhelpful or dangerous;

- expression of feelings varies between cultures and less expression does not necessarily mean abnormal psychology;

- most research studies have found psychodynamic approaches to be the least effective.

(Milner and O'Byrne 2009: 98–9)

Further exploration: deepening and understanding

After obtaining a broad overview of psychosocial work from these core texts the next stage in systematically collecting data is to return to the texts and identify key authors cited by the writers. All three authors make reference to some of the original work in the 1960s and 1970s (Hollis 1964, 1970; Hollis and Woods 1981). If you wish to learn more about the origins of the psychosocial case work, then you could return to those texts. Returning to original texts can be very rewarding as they provide detailed consideration of techniques that can be used in psychosocial case work. In terms of the developments of psychosocial casework, attachment theory is discussed by two authors (Payne 2005; Milner and O'Byrne 2009). To further an understanding of this, references to the work of key attachment theorists, for example, Bowlby (1963, 1979, 1982, 1988), Ainsworth *et al.* (1978) and Howe (1995, 2000), should be followed up, and recent research identified. Psychosocial work's potential for being oppressive is central to the critiques of all three authors and so, for example, references to the pathologising of black service users (Dominelli 2008) might be followed up.

 As I suggest in Chapter 4, in addition to building on the references supplied by the authors, an electronic search of databases will produce results which will identify other compendium textbooks, specialised textbooks and articles. This will provide more material on psychosocial work in general and, if you are looking for material with regard to specific service user groups, key words will refine the search.

Task-centred approach

Origins, theoretical underpinnings and core principles

Task-centred social work was developed in the 1970s in North America (Reid and Shyne 1969; Reid and Epstein 1972; Reid 1978) and in the 1970s and 1980s in the UK (Goldberg *et al.* 1985), at a time when longer-term therapeutic work based on the psychosocial method, discussed above, was the dominant form of social work. Reid and Shyne (1969) developed the brief casework approach following a four-year research study in a voluntary agency in which service users were offered either a 'traditional' longer-term service, usually lasting up to eighteen months, or a brief service of eight interviews. Their analysis of the outcomes found that improvement in the problems presented were greater in those families receiving the shorter-term intervention, and in some cases the longer-term intervention resulted in the family circumstances deteriorating. Following this a more refined task-centred method was developed (Reid and Epstein 1972). In the UK Goldberg *et al.* (1985) demonstrated that the approach was applicable to work in the statutory context of social services department teams in England. In research with two 'intake' or reception teams, a probation department and a hospital department, the approach was found to be suitable in two-thirds of cases. There has been more recent development of the task-centred approach in the UK by Doel and Marsh (Doel and Marsh 1992; Marsh and Doel 2005).

Reid (1972) argues that there is no underlying theoretical base for task-centred practice. Coulshed and Orme (2006) suggest that the theories underlying task-centred practice are only 'concepts' which include the notion of 'crisis' (Coulshed and Orme 2006: 166). Although a specific theoretical base cannot be identified, the approach is based on notions such as crisis, working with motivation, building on strengths, and 'step-by-step' problem solving. Payne (2005) argues that the approach is influenced by social learning theory, with the emphasis on the identification of targets and tasks, and rehearsal of action; communication theory, in respect of the emphasis on the sequencing and interacting behaviours; cognitive theory, with the concern about addressing beliefs of service users; and systems theory, given the location of service user problems in the wider environment. He draws interesting comparisons between task-centred approaches and crisis intervention. Milner and O'Byrne (2009) also identify that the task-centred approach is influenced by both cognitive theory and crisis intervention approaches (Parad 1965).

In summary, task-centred practice is short and time-limited intervention. It is suggested that between eight and twelve interviews take place between the service user and the social worker. It involves the social worker assisting the service user to identify the most important problems achievable within the time scale. The emphasis is on the development of small tasks which can be undertaken by the service user alone, tandem tasks undertaken by the service user and other parties, or joint tasks. The aim is to build on service user motivation by the incremental achievement of tasks. The skills learned in task completion can then be transferred by the service user to other areas of their lives. The termination of the piece of work is a key element in the success of task-centred work.

The processes and techniques of task-centred social work

The process of task-centred work involves problem classification; goal setting; task identification; and termination. With regard to problem classification, the task-centred approach has been found to be suitable for work in eight problem areas:

1. interpersonal conflict;

2. dissatisfaction in social relations;

3. problems with formal organisations;

4. difficulties in role performance;

5. problems of social transition;

6. reactive emotional distress;

7. inadequate resources (Reid 1978);

8. behavioural problems (Reid and Hanrahan 1981).

Milner and O'Byrne (2009), building on the development of the method by the authors Doel and Marsh (1992, 2005), provide a useful synthesis of the stages of task-centred work, and identify assessment questions which relate to six stages of the process. These are summarised below.

Stage 1: Meeting the service user

The social worker would need to know if the service user was self-referred or referred by a third party and issues of identification of need and mandatory referral explored.

Stage 2: Exploring the wants

The social worker would explore the needs or wants of the service user and find out if the service user wants a service. There is also a preliminary exploration of the causes of the problem.

Stage 3: Problem classification

The problem/s would be classified according to Reid's (1978) and Reid and Hanrahan's (1981) classification system. Interconnectedness between problems would be explored.

Stage 4: Agreeing a goal or goals

The focus would be on the specificity and achievability of goals with identification of changes, constraints and time scales.

Stage 5: Agreeing a task or tasks

In this stage tasks would be identified and agreement reached on who would carry these out.

Stage 6: Task implementation

During the implementation of tasks, ways in which task completion could be helped would be explored, for example through skill rehearsal or provision of resources.

Stage 7: Evaluation

A thorough review of task achievement would be undertaken and, if some were not achieved, the reasons identified. These reasons may be related to the service user, the social worker or the suitability of the tasks themselves.

This 'checklist' assists social workers in ensuring that they undertake task-centred social work in a critically reflective way, rather than approaching the work as a purely technical activity.

A range of techniques which can be used in each stage of the process have been identified by Coulshed and Orme (2006) which include: assisting the service user to ventilate and articulate the range of problems; negotiating the specific problems to be worked on and goals to be achieved, and identifying the tasks to be completed, and by whom; supporting task completion by referring to other support agencies, demonstrating and rehearsing skills; reviewing progress and facilitating task evaluation and review. Reid and Epstein (1972) highlight that workers need to develop the skills of *systematic* communication, which focuses on task completion and avoids attention drifting away from the identified problem, and those of *responsive* communication. Responsive communication involves the ability to address new issues which emerge during the work and to identify whether initial goals/tasks need to be revised.

Critical commentaries on task-centred case work

The authors of these three key texts in social work theory and practice have identified the following benefits and concerns of task-centred social work. Below are summaries of their key points.

Advantages and benefits:

- it offers clear accountability and an outcome focus approach for workers;

- the clarity of process and partnership working is welcomed by service users, and contributes to anti-oppressive practice;

- research supports the effectiveness of working with people in a focused way in a short time scale.
  (Payne 2005: 101, 116–17)

- a well-researched, feasible and effective approach, tried in a range of settings with a variety of service users, which offers a specific set of procedures;

- can take into account collective, as well as individual, experiences;

- the service user is the main change agent and the worker is a resource consultant;

- it encourages clarity of roles and purpose, and explicit statements of the social worker's account-ability and thereby avoids ambiguity;

- it offers the potential for the development of anti-oppressive practice as the agreement for work is open and the worker is accountable;

- practical advice is offered which can be modelled and rehearsed;

- the emphasis is on strengths and resources so it builds motivation and self-esteem;

- self-disclosure of service user to worker in a one-way vertical relationship is not required.

(Coulshed and Orme 2006: 169–72)

- suitable for any acknowledged problem which is capable of being solved by the service user with assistance;

- the service user defines the problem and is involved in task selection and completion;

- assists in developing service users' confidence if social workers are actively involved in assisting the completion of tasks alongside the service user;

- service users have the opportunity to demonstrate capacities as well as needs at early stages of the intervention;

- can result in social workers being more accountable, resulting in a more empowering and collab-orative approach;

- given the emphasis on service user involvement it may be less Eurocentric than other approaches.

(Milner and O'Byrne 2009: 136–8)

Disadvantages and concerns:

- not effective where consistent crises or long-term psychological issues are present;

- does not work well if the service user does not acknowledge the right of the service to be involved in their lives;

- the approach may be viewed by social workers in a simplistic way;

- the emphasis on individual problem solving means that the approach could mirror a medical rather than a social model of understanding situations;

- the use of contracts offers a false sense of equity between service users and workers and masks issue of power;

- it could be seen as providing a minimal response to severe social problems.

(Payne 2005: 116–17)

- task-centred practice may encourage workers to pigeonhole service users into having particular problems which fit into the method;

- it could lead to a form of behaviour modification;

- the method might be used to meet targets to reduce service provision and costs;

- rigid time limits will not be appropriate in all cases and may possibly ignore certain ethnic traditions.

(Coulshed and Orme 2006: 171–3)

- may sometimes not be appropriate, for example where service users have a mental health issue or are misusing drugs or alcohol;

- if used too rigidly, and without other approaches, it may be too narrow an approach;

- not suitable for long-standing, complex, existential problems;

- if viewed as intrinsically value free and anti-oppressive, it may lull social workers into not being continually aware of issues of oppression;

- social workers may become over-directive in their coaching role;

- no substantial evidence of the use of the approach with groups and communities.

(Milner and O'Byrne 2009: 136–8)

Further exploration: deepening an understanding

Following the process outlined in the above discussion of psychosocial work of how to further learning and deepen understanding, and after obtaining a broad overview of task-centred social work from the core texts, the next stage in systematically collecting data is to return to the texts and identify key authors cited by the writers. All three authors trace the origins of task-centred work in the United States to Reid (1978), Reid and Epstein (1972), and Reid and Shyne (1969), and, in the UK, to Goldberg et al. (1985). Returning to key texts can be very rewarding. The findings of empirical research and original case examples are provided. Very detailed information is given on the micro processes within each stage of task-centred case work, for example in defining the kinds of task which may be used. The more recent work of Doel and Marsh (1992) and Marsh and Doel (2005) are referred to by all three authors. These texts are modern-day classics which dedicate the entire volume to an exploration of task-centred work, and so provide in-depth analysis and detailed guidance. The critiques of the method can be further explored by initially pursuing references which are cited in the three core texts, for example with regard to black perspectives (Ahmad 1990; Devore and Schlesinger 1991).

In addition to building on the references supplied by the authors, an electronic search of databases and relevant journals will provide more material on task-centred work in general, and key words will assist refining the search if you are looking for material regarding specific service user groups.

In this chapter, two social work methods have been introduced. You have been shown how a preliminary reading of a small number of core texts can provide an understanding of the origins, theoretical underpinnings, processes and techniques and critique of a method. Although these texts are very comprehensive it is important that you widen your reading to access different perspectives and ways of viewing social work methods of intervention. Advice has been given on how to develop learning and deepen your understanding of methods of intervention. In the next chapter we will provide a framework which will further assist both the critique of social work interventions and the consideration of how the written material on methods can be used in practice situations.

Exercise 1

Cognitive behavioural therapy is a well-researched and well-used method of social work intervention. Using the method and structure demonstrated above, identify three core social work texts other than the texts used in this chapter and summarise:

- the origins of cognitive behavioural therapy;

- theoretical underpinnings and core principles;

- processes and techniques;

- critical commentary;

- advantages and benefits;

- disadvantages and concerns;

- further exploration regarding deepening an understanding.

Exercise 2

Having undertaken the first exercise now choose a service user group and problem area and identify two pieces of cognitive behavioural research, which have been undertaken in that area, which might assist you to decide whether cognitive behavioural therapy might be the most appropriate intervention in that situation.

Key learning points

- A sound understanding of methods of intervention can be gained by a systematic reading of key texts.

- Differences of opinion among authors about methods of intervention may be slight at times but important to register.

- The initial reading should be supplemented with further reading advised by authors of key texts and through the research method given in Chapter 4 in order to further and deepen their understanding.

Further reading

Clark, A. (2007) 'Crisis intervention', in J. Lishman (ed.), *Handbook for practice learning in social care and social work*, 2nd edn, London: Jessica Kingsley.

Marsh, P. and Doel, M. (2005) *The task-centred book*, London: Routledge.

9 Furthering the critique and applying the method

In this chapter, we will first of all explore another tool which will assist in the development of critical analysis and the integration of theory and practice. This chapter builds on the previous chapter which outlined two methods of intervention and gave a basic critique of them. Here, I will introduce a Critical Analysis Framework (CAF) which was initially developed by students in the second year of the postgraduate social work course at the University of Glasgow to assist in their analysis of methods of intervention. After explaining how the framework was developed, a summary of students' evaluation of the framework will be provided to give some indications of the possible uses and purposes of a framework. A revised CAF, which has been updated to include concepts developed in more recent social work literature and to ensure that the framework is more suitable for use by students towards the beginning of their course, will be presented. The purpose of each element of the framework will be discussed before it is used to further critique a third method of intervention, solution-focused therapy.

The process of developing the Critical Analysis Framework

The framework was developed by students as part of a module which introduced students to social work methods. At the beginning of the module students were asked how they might be assisted to develop their skills of critical understanding of social work theory. We discussed the development of a framework which could serve as one tool of analysis. Students drew on their reading to develop the framework and then used this instrument throughout the module, as they were introduced to different social work methods of intervention. As the module progressed, students continued to develop the framework, which was further amended by students in workshops during their period of practice learning.

Evaluation of the use of the framework

The use of the framework was evaluated by students and tutors. Most students had found the framework useful in preparing for and writing their case or practice study. Students also found that the framework assisted them in critically analysing theory and integrating theory and practice while in placement:

> Overall it got me thinking about how to start critically analysing the models I was using.

> In a general sense it helped to break down thoughts about theories and form a more structured analysis.

> The framework helped me think more extensively about the use of theory in practice.

> I felt that I could investigate theory before I looked at it. However now I see that my way of choosing theories wasn't adequate and I have come to this conclusion through using the framework. I now feel that I am much more able to integrate theory and practice.

A particular benefit for students was the consideration of theoretical underpinnings of the method:

> It makes you think about the historical context and the purpose of the theory.

> I was prompted to look at the research behind each social work method, to see where it has been effective and where it hadn't.

> It provides a model for a general critical analysis of all theory in the assignment.

> In the course of my course work, I critically analysed some influential theories which influenced the way I wrote about these in my practice study.

Tutors echoed these views:

> The framework is useful for getting into the complexity of the application of a method. I think

it is too easy for students to glibly talk about, say, a task-centred approach, without considering fully what the application means. The framework allows students to consider all aspects of a model of intervention.

The inclusion of anti-oppressive practice principles is important as well, as students are being given the opportunity to consider dominant discourses informing models/methods of practice.

Here is a revised Critical Analysis Framework which might assist students to critically analyse theory in a structured way.

CRITICAL ANALYSIS FRAMEWORK

Theoretical underpinnings

What are the theoretical underpinnings of the method of intervention?

Research evidence of effectiveness

What is the research evidence which supports this method?

What is its effectiveness with regard to particular issues or service users?

Anti-oppressive practice

How does this method assist in the development of anti-oppressive practice?

How does it assist in an

- analysis of social difference;

- analysis of power?

Service user involvement

Has the method potential for empowerment of the service user?

How does the method promote service user and carer participation and involvement?

What particular skills are required in order for me to effectively use this method?

Personal value base

How does this method sit within my own value base and ethical principles?

Explaining the sections of the framework

Theoretical underpinnings

What are the theoretical underpinnings of the method of intervention?

In order to answer this question you will need to review a range of literature on the method. You will find that different writers hold different views as to theoretical underpinnings. As we saw in the last chapter, there may be disagreement as to the theoretical underpinnings of a method. For example, the original author of the task-centred method stated that it was theoryless (Reid 1972), while a later commentator (Payne 2005) has argued that task-centred social work draws on the theoretical principles of learning theory, communication theory and systems theory.

Identifying what you consider to be the theoretical underpinnings of a method of intervention is the start of developing your critique of the method. It is going back to the foundations of the method, as you are beginning to question what the proponents of the method, and commentators on the method, view as the core principles of understanding.

Research evidence of effectiveness

What is the research evidence which supports this method?

What is its effectiveness with regard to particular issues or service users?

These questions prompt you to consider the evidence for the effectiveness of the social work method in particular agencies and service user situations. This requires you to return to the core compendium textbooks in order to gain an overview of research, and then to seek out relevant examples of original research and research overviews. As Payne (2005) discusses, there is limited evidence of the effectiveness of particular social work methods. Task-centred practice, behavioural social work, family therapy and cognitive behavioural social work do have a body of research literature in the health and social work fields. There is also evaluation research which evaluates a particular agency approach or policy, for example family group conferencing in child care social work (Barnsdale and Walker 2007) or pro-social modelling in probation practice (Trotter 2006). However, although examination of a practice method may be part of this kind of evaluation research, social work methods, as discussed in this text, may not be specifically evaluated. Also, there is very little comparison of the effectiveness of methods of intervention (Payne 2005). Where research evidence is limited, students need to acknowledge that, and use other areas of the CAF to assist them in choosing an appropriate method of intervention for the service user's situation.

Anti-oppressive practice

How does this method assist in the development of anti-oppressive practice?

How does it assist in an

- analysis of social difference;
- analysis of power?

These questions invite you to consider how explicitly the method addresses issues of social difference. Does the method have the potential, intentionally or otherwise, to homogenise or pathologise service users? For example, it has been argued that a cognitive behavioural approach to social work is based on evidence of good outcomes and is a transparent, value-free approach, as goals and interventions are open and explicit (Sheldon 2000). However, behavioural social work has been criticised on the basis of being 'largely psychologically reductionist', that is, based on a simplistic understanding of human beings in their psychological and social situations (Milner and O'Byrne 2009: 119). This would suggest that behavioural approaches may be criticised for not recognising difference. Psychosocial approaches have been valued in that they encourage an open-minded, reflexive, accepting approach (Coulshed and Orme 2006), but the value base of these approaches has been questioned in respect of the potential to pathologise or to blame the victim (Payne 2005). The explicit construction of the social worker as the expert in the process also questions the potential of the method to address the inherent power imbalance in the relationship between the social worker and the service user.

Service user involvement

Has the method potential for empowerment of the service user?

How does the method promote service user and carer participation and involvement?

It could be argued that all methods have the potential to promote service user participation and involvement to some extent. A service user may be consulted about the use of a particular method of intervention, for example a choice between a talking therapy such as counselling, cognitive behavioural therapy, or group therapy. However, some methods of intervention could be considered to be more intrinsically empowering than others. For example, the explicitness of the task-centred process, with the focus on the service user involvement in determining the most pressing problems and identifying tasks, has been viewed as potentially empowering (Milner and O'Byrne 2009), although there is an unresolved debate with regard to the empowering nature of the use of contracts in the method (Corden and Preston-Shoot 1987, 1988; Rojek and Collins 1987, 1988).

Skills

What particular skills are required in order for me to effectively use this method?

The effectiveness of a method is also dependent on the skills of the social worker at that moment in time. You need to be aware of the skills required in implementing a method and how you might begin to develop those skills through training and practice.

Personal value base

How does this method sit within my own value base and ethical principles?

Student social workers enter social work courses with more or less explicit values and ethical beliefs. These may be drawn from personal experience, education, religious background and beliefs, political beliefs and professional understanding of ethical issues. In considering the use of a method of intervention, personal values are likely to impact on decisions about which to use. An explicit discussion of this is important in developing the capacity to reflect, involving intellectual, effective activity which can result in different perspectives on issues.

Implementing the framework: solution-focused therapy

Theoretical underpinnings

What are the theoretical underpinnings of the method/model?

It has been argued by the founders of solution-focused therapy that it is atheoretical (de Shazer 1985, 1988, 1991, 1994). However, other commentators suggest that the method is influenced by post-modernism and social constructionism in that it rejects dominant discourses of professional expertise in solving people's problems, but suggests, instead, that there are multiple understandings of situations, and that service users have the expertise to find their own solutions (Milner and O'Byrne 2009). The approach can be understood by exploring the key tenets of social constructionism in which it is understood that there are multiple interpretations of the 'truth' of any situation. Perspectives on any situation are dependent on social and political contexts and meanings are constructed through language (Parton and O'Byrne 2000). Social workers working from a social constructivist paradigm would therefore acknowledge that they are working with uncertainty, or 'working truths'. Solution-focused therapy shares similar theoretical underpinning with other therapies working from a strengths perspective (Healy 2005). Like other strengths-perspective approaches, solution-focused therapy rejects psychoanalytic theory-based approaches, which concentrate on long-term counselling in respect of problems and which focus on insight into the past, as it is considered that this can lead to an over-emphasis on deficiencies and blaming behaviours (O'Connell 1998). Milner and O'Byrne (2009) suggest solution-focused therapy is mainly a cognitive approach which concentrates on the actions of the service user rather than the intervention of the professionals. It has similarities with narrative therapy in that it differentiates the problem from the person and names the problem as a consequence of social processes and not of individual failings. Likewise, the emphasis on finding solutions is based on emphasising differences and exceptions to the problem.

Research evidence of effectiveness

What is the research evidence which supports this method?

What is its effectiveness with regard to particular issues or service users?

Research carried out by de Shazer at the Milwaukee Brief Family Therapy Center in the United States provides evidence for the efficacy of the approach (de Shazer 1985, 1988). Gingerich and Eisenhart (2000) undertook a systematic review of outcome studies in the field of solution-focused therapy. A systematic review is a review of the literature which investigates a particular research area by identifying research studies, critically evaluating the rigour of the methodology and validity of the findings of those studies, usually to pre-determined criteria, and making judgement about the quality of the research. Gingerich and Eisenhart (2000) identified five *well-controlled* studies in which positive outcomes were evident in work with depressed students, parenting skills, rehabilitation of orthopaedic patients and recidivism in prisons. The European Brief Therapy Association (n.d.) found that the success of the intervention in forty-seven outcome studies, rated by service users themselves, was high in the areas of anorexia, violence, drug misuse, and mental health. They found no difference in outcomes with regard to the age, gender or ethnicity of the service user.

However, Payne (1995) argues that although solution-focused therapy has been well-evaluated in its initial trials, and has become an accepted and well-used approach in social work practice, 'its formal implementation in social work settings has not led to research to validate it as a theory' (Payne 1995: 53). In a similar vein, Corcoran and Pillai (2009) argue that there are few valid evaluations of the success of the method. In their systematic evaluation of outcome studies, they found that the effectiveness of the approach was 'equivocal and more rigorously designed research needs to establish its effectiveness. Therefore, practitioners should understand there is not a strong evidence basis for solution-focused therapy at this point in time' (Corcoran and Pillai 2009: 240). Clearly a key issue here is what approach to evaluation is taken, for example service user feedback or controlled trials. This raises questions with regard to qualitative and quantitative research methods and ethical issues in research. Shaw, Briar-Lawson, Orme and Ruckdeschel (2010) provide a very comprehensive overview of social work research.

Anti-oppressive practice

How does this method accord with the following anti-oppressive principles:

- analysis of social difference;

- analysis of power?

Solution-focused therapy is concerned with *difference* in the postmodern sense of the word. It does not emphasise structurally constructed social differences, but rather differences in and between individual and dominant discourses. Solution-focused therapy seeks to disrupt the dominant professional and other discourses by privileging the service user perspective. The analysis of power takes place at the level of the therapeutic encounter and is concerned with the relationship between the service user and the social worker, where the service user's reality is the central focus. However, concern has been expressed that solution-focused therapy can ignore, or appear to ignore, structural power relations such as gender (Dermer *et al.* 1998).

Service user involvement

Has the method potential for empowerment of the service user?

How does the method promote service user and carer participation and involvement?

Solution-focused therapy takes a critical theory approach to the social construction of problems, with the aim of service user empowerment. Solution-focused therapy proponents argue against established long-term therapeutic interventions in favour of a more radical, short-term, social constructionist approach (de Shazer 1985, 1988). Therapists using a solution-focused approach argue that the service user is the expert on their own problems, and has the power and ability to find solutions to those problems. A social worker using solution-focused therapy would not become involved in interpreting situations on behalf of the service user in the position of an expert.

Solution-focused therapy takes a future-orientated perspective. The social worker using solution-focused therapy enters the relationship with the service user with no assumptions with regard to the problem, the service user's past, how things might change, or what the solutions might be. The social worker does not impose a meaning on the service users' talk (Myers 2007). Solution-focused therapy argues for the legitimacy, indeed the paramountcy, of the service user's perspective.

Skills

What particular skills are required in order for me to effectively use this method?

O'Connell (2005) offers the following practice guidance for practitioners planning to use solution-focused therapy:

- Use every session with a client, including the first, as if it were the last.

- Project confidence and hope that much can be achieved in a limited time.

- Stay close to the client's agenda.

- Trust the competence of your client and keep out of his or her way.

- Ask yourself what difference would it make to your practice if you really believed that more is not better, better is better.

- Consider ways of evaluating your work.

(O'Connell 2005: 6)

Solution-focused therapy relies on the skill of listening, as the aim is to hear the service user's views on their own solutions. Social workers using this method must develop the skills of assisting the service user to focus on the problem-free moment, on interruptions to the problem and to focus on the future. Social workers need to avoid dwelling on the problem, looking to past causes, and attempting to interpret the problem and suggest solutions. This is a challenge when social workers have been trained and are working using problem-solving approaches.

Milner and O'Byrne provide an excellent overview of practice techniques employed in solution-focused therapy (2009: 146–52). They identify the use of simple questions, miracle questions, scaled questions and coping questions. The miracle question is set up to assist the service user to imagine what it would be like in a problem-free future. The formula would be to ask a service user to imagine that a miracle happened and the problems had disappeared. They are asked to consider what would be different and if any of those different things exist already. Scaled questions are likely to be framed as: 'On a scale of one to ten, how depressed/anxious/angry do you feel at the moment?' The aim of this kind of question is to detach the problem from the person and assist the person to consider the problem as an entity outside the service user, which is open to change. This is in order to emphasise the exceptions to the existing problem. After a solution-focused framing of the situation has been established, the setting of future-focused tasks takes place alongside the service user, with the service user determining the most appropriate tasks, experimenting, and recording differences which develop as a result of the task. The ability to give oral and written feedback to facilitate the service user in finding her or his own solutions is also a core skill.

Personal value base

How does this method sit within my own value base and ethical principles?

Solution-focused therapy may challenge aspects of your personal and professional values and ethical principles. How comfortable are you with being future-focused and not exploring the past when you yourself may have benefited from counselling which encouraged and challenged you to examine past experiences, with a beneficial effect? Do you have political views with regard to analysing structural dimensions of power?

Practice example

Sara is a twenty-year-old woman who has contacted social services. She is white and not disabled. In an initial interview Sara gives you a brief background to why she has approached social services. Sara has previously lived rough on the streets and in homeless hostel accommodation. She is a drug user and has been involved in prostitution in the past to support her and her partner's habits. She and her partner are now on a methadone programme. However, Sara has begun to use heroin again. Her partner has started to become orally abusive to Sara and had threatened to throw her out if she continues to use. Sara says that she wishes to stay with her partner as she has nowhere else to go. She indicates that for most of the time her partner is not abusive and he is aware that she has come to social services. He has indicated that he is struggling to cope with remaining heroin-free. Sara states: 'It's my fault he's getting angry with me. He's trying to stay off and he says I'm encouraging him to start using again. I'm not. It's just my way of coping when I get a bit down.'

Consider that you might be allocated this case whilst in a reception team, or equivalent, in a statutory social work department. What might solution-focused therapy have to offer in this situation?

Theoretical underpinnings

What would a social constructionist approach have to offer in this situation? Work with Sara would be based on an understanding that there are multiple understandings of the situation. Sara herself might have contradictory views with regard to her own substance misuse and the potential developing abuse from her partner. The partner brings other perspectives to the situation. A social constructionist approach would pay attention to the language or discourse used by Sara to describe her situation.

Research evidence of effectiveness

There is some research evidence that suggest that solution-focused therapy has been found to be effective in areas of substance misuse and interpersonal violence (Gingerich and Eisenhart 2000). However, the precise nature of this evidence would need to be ascertained, for example, what types of drug misuse does the research address and in which settings did the research take place? Milner and O'Byrne (2009) discuss how a solution-focused approach would concentrate on safety rather than risks. Milner (2008a, 2008b) shows how solution-focused therapy can be used where there is violence in interpersonal relationships. However, this research focuses on the person who is perpetrating the violence. If Sara's partner agrees to become involved in therapy, might this be useful? If he does not, might this nevertheless offer alternative perspectives on the situation? What evidence is there for the use of solution-focused therapy with victims/survivors of abuse, for example sexual abuse, given Sara has been involved in prostitution? From whose perspective is the evidence drawn? As well as 'well-controlled' clinical trial evidence, is there 'softer' evidence, drawn from service users and social workers, which could be investigated?

Anti-oppressive practice

A solution-focused approach would understand power as a postmodern concept, with emphasis on difference. The social worker would make no assumptions with regard to Sara's past experiences, problems and solutions. Sara's perspective would be privileged in the sessions. Instead of concentrating on past experiences as a victim of abuse to gain insight into the problem, Sara would be encouraged to consider exceptions and she would be assisted to explore how different power relationships could exist in the future. However, concern has been expressed that solution-focused therapy ignores structural power differences such as gender, for example in cases of domestic violence (Dermer *et al.* 1998).

Service user perspectives

The social worker would adopt a 'not-knowing' stance in relation to Sara's experiences and understandings. Sara's views of her experience would be seen as paramount. The emphasis of the work would be to facilitate Sara into determining her own solutions to the issue of substance misuse and domestic abuse. The worker would not impose their views on how to solve Sara's issues. On the one hand, offering no advice may be difficult for workers who have experience in working with people who misuse drugs and are aware of the long-term effects of substance misuse. On the other hand, workers may be being aware of the likelihood of relapse in recovery from substance misuse and may wish to share the experiences of others with Sara, to encourage her in her attempts to be heroin-free. This knowledge is background knowledge which informs the worker's approach, however Sara's situation should be viewed as unique. In the discussion of anti-oppressive practice, feminist concerns with regard to the use of solution-focused therapy in situations of domestic abuse were highlighted. However, solution-focused therapy is not incompatible with feminist approaches in cases of domestic abuse. Leaving a domestic abuse situation is a process which may be reflected upon and then planned well in advance of leaving (Barron 2009 for Women's Aid). Should Sara decide to leave the relationship at a future date, based on her own assessment of the situation and ways of resolving issues, solution-focused therapy could then complement the guidance from Women's Aid.

Skills

The skills needed in working with Sara would be based on ensuring that the focus of the work is on listening to Sara's perspective, whilst encouraging her to be future-focused. The worker would be projecting confidence, verbally and non-verbally, that Sara had the ability to decide on changes that would help eliminate the problem and the competence to achieve the solutions. Questions used to assist Sara in this would include the use of a miracle question, asking her what her life would be like if the problem no longer existed. Sara could be asked to scale her anxiety in order to externalise the problem.

Personal value base

The worker may feel ethically comfortable in using solution-focused therapy with Sara, as the focus is on Sara's perspectives and Sara's strengths. The worker's value base may also be challenged. Concern for Sara's safety may raise ethical issues for the worker. The possible risk to Sara from the substance misuse and the domestic violence may lead them to think that solution-focused therapy is not an appropriate method of intervention in this case.

In this chapter a Critical Analysis Framework has been introduced to assist you to critically analyse theory and to integrate theory and practice. The elements of the framework were explored before it was applied to one method of intervention, solution-focused therapy. This method was chosen because students can find it to be a conceptually difficult method to understand. The framework can assist you to break down different elements of the method to assist understanding. The framework can be added to or adapted by you to meet your particular learning needs.

Exercise 1

Stefan is twenty-six and came to the UK from Poland four years ago to work in the building industry. He was made unemployed nine months ago. Stefan lives with his partner Darren, thirty-two, who is British. Darren works casually in bar work, but he is in employment most of the time. The men live in a furnished rented apartment in the city centre. The apartment is in poor repair, with two broken windows and poor heating facilities. The letting agency have been informed and have said they have alerted the owner but no action has been taken. In the last three months Stefan has become depressed and has visited his GP who has diagnosed mild depression and prescribed anti-depressants. In the last two weeks the two men have been subject to oral abuse by neighbours. Some of this is in respect of the poor condition of the flat and some in respect of their being in a gay relationship. Stefan comes to the social work agency for assistance.

Using the Critical Analysis Framework develop a critical analysis of how a crisis intervention approach to social work intervention might be used in respect of the above service user.

> **Exercise 2**
>
> - What have you found the most useful and least useful elements in the framework?
> - Consider what elements you would add to the framework and why.
> - Are there any existing areas that you would not include?

Key learning points

- The critical analysis of social work methods of intervention can be assisted by adopting a systematic approach as demonstrated in the case study.

- Highlighting anti-oppressive practice and service user and carer involvement in any framework ensures that these aspects of the critique are not omitted.

- Students can construct their own framework which aids their critical analysis and integrating of theory and practice.

Further reading

Myers, J. (2007) *Theory into practice: Solution-focused approaches*, Lyme Regis: Russell House.

O'Connell, B. (2005) *Solution-focused therapy*, 2nd edn, London: Sage.

10 Critical Incident Analysis

Critical Incident Analysis is a tool which is being used increasingly in social work education. This chapter will describe the origins of Critical Incident Analysis and provide definitions of the approach. It will give examples of a range of uses for Critical Incident Analysis, by students and service users, before introducing one developed by myself and Dr Beth R. Crisp (Green Lister and Crisp 2007). Students' views of using Critical Incident Analysis will be given, as well as one student's Critical Incident Analysis and her evaluation of it. The focus of the use of the framework is on students' experiences in practice learning.

The origins of Critical Incident Analysis

Critical Incident Analysis was first developed in the aviation industry and in anaesthesia in order to analyse near-misses, pilot errors and complications in the operating theatre. This form of Critical Incident Analysis was concerned with assessing risk. The aim was to look at failures of procedures or human error to ensure that similar mistakes were not repeated. Critical Incident Analysis has been used in fields related to social work, particularly health, over the last twenty years, for example in nursing and midwifery (Rich and Parker 1995) and mental health nursing (Minghella and Benson 1995).

What is a critical incident?

There are a number of definitions of critical incidents. Here are two influential authors' definitions of a critical incident.

> The vast majority of critical incidents . . . are not all dramatic or obvious; they are straightforward accounts of very commonplace events that occur in routine professional practice which are critical in the rather different sense that they are indicative of underlying trends, motives and structures. These incidents appear to be 'typical' rather than 'critical' at first sight but are rendered critical through analysis.
>
> (Tripp 1993: 24–5)

In brief a critical incident is any occurrence which was significant to a person for whatever reason. It may have been important because it was traumatic, or even because it was so mundane that it encapsulated something crucial about the nature of their work. It may have been remembered because it is unresolved, or posed a dilemma for the person. It may have struck a high point for them, or marked a turning point in their thinking. 'It is important to remember that the "incident" should be a description of something concrete, rather than a more abstract issue or situation' (Fook 2002: 98–9).

As can be seen from the above quotations, Critical Incident Analysis in social work and social work education is not necessarily concerned with a dramatic incident such as a 'near miss' in aviation but rather as an event which caused a person to 'stop and think' either during or after an event. An example of a critical incident might well be when a student is working with an older person who then dies, or when a student is inadvertently involved in a case of child protection, and these could be analysed through the Critical Incident Analysis. However, the incident could be the recognition of underlying trends as suggested by Tripp (1993). These could be positive, an awareness of the support given you by another student, which you realise that you had taken for granted, or negative, being aware in a workplace that a much-disliked task was always left for you to do. Critical incidents may be a 'high point' suggested by Fook (2002: 99). Positive feedback from a service user could be an example of this.

The development of Critical Incident Analysis in social work

In social work education, within and outside the UK, different forms of Critical Incident Analysis have been used to assist students and service users in the development of critical reflection. Four examples of research into the use of Critical Incident Analysis are given below.

CASE EXAMPLE 1

Social work students and service users: ethnoracial identity (Montalvo 1999)

Students at the University of Texas were asked to conduct Critical Incident Interviews with service users. The aims of the interviews were to assess the service users' understandings of their ethnoracial identity. Students interviewed someone from a different racial group about the critical incidents in their lives which influenced their ethnoracial identity. Following the interviews, students produced a narrative report and presented findings in a classroom discussion. The students found that by discussing how critical incidents had affected service users' understanding of their ethnoracial identity, the service users were able to develop a coherent narrative of what ethnoracial identity meant for them. In addition, following the discussion of the interviews with service users, social work students submitted their own Critical Incident Analysis of how the interviews had increased their own cultural awareness and improved their intellectual grasp of identity formation.

CASE EXAMPLE 2

Social work students: intercultural understanding (Legault 1996)

Critical Incident Analysis was used here to address the culture shock faced by social work students in Quebec, Canada in their first period of practice learning. Critical Incident Interviews were carried out with social work students to assist them to analyse situations of intercultural understanding.

CASE EXAMPLE 3

Critical Incident Analysis as assessment of practice (Monash University n.d.)

Students in Monash University in Australia were required to use Critical Incident Analysis as part of the assessment of their practice. Students were required to:

- consider an incident which was crucial to or significant to their learning;

- reflect on the incident with regard to its impact on their beliefs and values on action;

- consider its impact on the development of professional judgement.

CASE EXAMPLE 4

Critical Incident Analysis in supervision when in practice learning (Davies and Kinloch 2000: 140)

A Critical Incident Analysis tool was developed by practice teachers in Scotland to assist students to critically reflect in supervision. In order to assist students to consider both positive and negative experiences students were asked to select one incident which was significant to them and to bring it to supervision. The following suggestions for choice of incidents were given:

- when you felt you had done something well;

- when you had made the wrong decision;

- when something went better than expected;

- when you lacked confidence;

- when you made a mistake;

- when you really enjoyed working with someone or a group;

- when you had a feeling of pressure;

- when you found it difficult to accept or value a service user/s;

- when you realised you did not know enough;

- when you felt unsupported.

Students were then asked to make brief notes to take to supervision with regard to the points in respect of: description of the event, putting the event in context, their role in the event, the purpose and focus of intervention, how they thought and felt about the event, reminders of previous experience or learning, feelings and thoughts about the outcome, learning (about self, relationships, social work task, organisation, procedures, what they might do differently), issues of reflection to take to supervision.

The four examples show the variety of ways that Critical Incident Analysis can be used. In the first example students asked service users to consider a critical incident and then interviewed them about this. In social work education Critical Incident Analysis appears to be used mainly in written form, where a series of questions are given to students or practitioners, and written responses are made. However, an oral account of a critical incident could be given. If, for example the discussion of the critical incident was part of an ongoing assessment process between a practice teacher and a student, it would be useful if the student had advance notice of the particular questions to be asked, as illustrated in the example from Davies and Kinloch (2000) above, so that they could reflect on their responses. The same would apply to the use of oral Critical Incident Analysis with service users.

In the university or whilst in practice learning, Critical Incident Analysis may be used in an ongoing way to encourage reflection, criticality and professional development as in the examples from Montalvo (1999), Legault (1996) and Davies and Kinloch (2000). They may also be used as part of the formal assessment process as in the example from Monash University (n.d.).

Fook (2002) has been highly influential in developing the theoretical base and educational tools for critical incident technique. She suggests that social workers should develop a detailed written descriptive story of an incident. She then offers a series of nine questions for social workers to answer which would assist them to construct and deconstruct the critical incident. This technique requires a sophisticated understanding of critical theory and critical deconstruction and reconstruction. I would suggest that students in the latter stages of their social work education use Fook's (2002) tool to further develop their skills of critical reflection. However, for students who are near the beginning of their social work education, I suggest that the Critical Incident Analysis tool developed by Green Lister and Crisp (2007), and presented below, is a useful starting point.

CRITICAL INCIDENT ANALYSIS FRAMEWORK

Account of the incident

- What happened, where and when? Who was involved?

- What was your role/involvement in the incident?

- What was the context of this incident, e.g. previous involvement of yourself or others from this agency with this client/client group?

- What was the purpose and focus of your contact/intervention at this point?

Initial responses to the incident

- What were your thoughts and feelings at the time of this incident?

- What were the responses of other key individuals to this incident? If not known, what do you think these might have been?

Issues and dilemmas highlighted by this incident

- What practice dilemmas were identified as a result of this incident?

- What are the values and ethical issues which are highlighted by this incident?

- Are there implications for inter-disciplinary and/or inter-agency collaborations which you have identified as a result of this incident?

Learning

- What have you learned, e.g. about yourself, relationships with others, the social work task, organisational policies, and procedures?

- What theory (or theories) has (or might have) helped develop your understanding about some aspect of this incident?

- What research has (or might have) helped develop your understanding about some aspect of this incident?

- How might an understanding of the legislative, organisational and policy contexts explain some aspects associated with this incident?

- What future learning needs have you identified as a result of this incident? How might this be achieved?

Outcomes

- What were the outcomes of this incident for the various participants?

- Are there ways in which this incident has led (or might lead to) changes in how you think, feel or act in particular situations?

- What are your thoughts and feelings now about this incident?

The *account* of the incident concentrates on the facts of the incident. The questions are asking you to describe the incident at this point and not to reflect or analyse it.

The section on *initial responses* to the incident aims to assist you to remember your immediate thoughts but also feelings. You are asked to comment on the reaction of others. The focus here is still on description, although the questions invite you to begin reflection on thoughts and feelings.

The questions with regard to *issues and dilemmas* direct you to consider value and ethical issues. Here you may wish to reflect on issues such as anti-oppressive practice. The dilemmas you discuss may be those related specifically to the incident or may be about future dilemmas that you anticipate that you will face as a result of the incident. There are no 'why' questions in the framework. This is intentional as 'why' questions asked by others can at times be unhelpfully confrontational. If the incident that you wish to discuss is one where you feel that you did not handle a situation very well, then a 'why' question might lead to a consideration of blame.

The section on *learning* is the most complex, and consequently will probably take the longest time to complete. The questions ask you to consider personal learning that you can take from the incident in a number of areas. Not all the areas may be relevant to the incident you are discussing so you will be choosing those which are the most significant for you. Similarly, the question on legal and organisational contexts may be very or only tangentially relevant to the particular incident which you are discussing. You are asked to consider theories and research which had or might have assisted you in developing your understanding. Here, it would be useful to ask yourself the 'why' question as this requires you to go into more depth in considering the theory. Merely naming a theory or an author would not allow you to demonstrate your understanding of the relationship between theory and practice.

The section on outcomes asks you to state the outcomes for all participants. You might wish to reflect on whether these were positive or negative outcomes for all the parties concerned.

How useful have students found Critical Incident Analysis?

The Critical Incident Analysis was piloted by ten students and their practice teachers. When on practice learning placement students were asked to produce a Critical Incident Analysis once a week for supervision. Midway through, and after the end of the placement, students were interviewed to ascertain their views on the use of the Critical Incident Analysis Framework on placement. Students were also asked to present an example of the Critical Incident Analysis at the interview and to talk through it. Practice assessors were also interviewed at the end of the placement.

Examples of situations where students used Critical Incident Analysis

The following four examples are from students who talked about the kinds of situations in which they had used Critical Incident Analysis. They show how it can be used in very different practice learning situations.

This first example is written by a student where the critical incident was when a visit to a service user when the student was concerned for her safety. This example is one which was written about a specific situation which had the potential to be dangerous.

> My last analysis was a home assessment visit I had to do where I was visiting a family where the father used methadone. I went to the house and the windows were painted over. I knocked on the door and the family asked me to go around the back and they locked the door when I went in. I thought about what we had discussed about safety in [Social Work Theory and Practice Module]. I was just about to ask him to unlock the door when he saw I was uncomfortable and apologised and asked me if I wanted it unlocked. I said yes and he did, saying it was just a habit. I used the framework to think through the dilemma.

In this second example it can be seen that the student is not writing about a specific one-off event but one where the student becomes aware that a service user has not been telling him the truth about his family situation. The student was working with the man in a facilitative way and faced a dilemma about telling his practice teacher about the incident. It caused the student to reflect on his statutory role.

> I used the framework with regard to a value dilemma in working with a men's group. The group was voluntary and my relationship with the men had been one of facilitating. However, when I was assisting one of the men to get funding for his child, it came to light that he had a recent history of drug and alcohol abuse and his children had been taken into care. I had to tell my practice teacher but felt very uncomfortable. I used the framework to help me consider the statutory role.

The third example is one where the student faces another ethical dilemma, but this time in relation to the attitudes of a co-worker.

> It was the second day of my placement and a co-worker made a racist remark. I knew I couldn't sit on it or that would be collusion so I used the framework to think it through and present to my practice teacher.

Extended example of a student's use of Critical Incident Analysis

This example begins with the written Critical Incident Analysis which the student gave to her practice teacher, followed by her evaluation of the use of the Critical Incident Analysis in that situation. This student was working with a child (CN) who was not attending school. The student had assessed the child's needs and was working with him and his mother with regard to his return to school.

Account of the incident

Discussion re CN with link worker. Link worker had received call to ask if he knew anyone who may benefit from an alternative to school place because there were still some free places. He suggested to me CN would be appropriate. This was unexpected as the plan was to review the situation once CN had returned to school.

Initial responses to the incident

I was unhappy with this because it didn't fit with my assessment of CN's needs and I argued strongly that this approach was inappropriate. I feel he is socially isolated but starting to make friends and taking him out of school would jeopardise this. I have identified that his mother's illness may be contributing to his isolation and have secured a consultation with the Child and Family Clinic to start addressing this. We haven't previously discussed with him alternatives to school as a realistic prospect and he clearly wants to stay in mainstream education. He has started the new term well and had attended every day so far so it seemed inappropriate to suddenly suggest an alternative to school. I was also aware of the impact a sudden decision like this could have on his mother's health.

I also felt that this proposal was service-led rather than needs-led. I felt really awkward because I was aware that it is unlikely a place in this service is likely to be readily available again. So I had to be confident of my assessment. On reflection I realise the theory I have used throughout my involvement with CN really helped me justify my position (see section 4).

Issues and dilemmas highlighted by this incident

It highlighted how the importance of listening to service users' views can be hindered by lack of resources, therefore, when resources become available staff can be over-eager to use them rather than lose them.

Learning

I used Trotter's [1999] framework while working with CN. He recommends using solution-focused approaches. I did so and this highlighted that CN recognised he is socially isolated and feels this is the main thing he wants to change. He also spoke about some elements of school being positive because he likes the subjects and his friends there. Because his mum doesn't let him out much this is the only time he has with his friends. I used this information to assess that he would lose these positive aspects if he was removed from school part of the week. Trotter

[1999] also recommends pro-social modelling and rewarding pro-social behaviour. I feel it would be really damaging not to recognise as positive his attempts to attend school during the first week back and that offering alternatives to school despite these efforts would be really negative. Because Trotter's [1999] approach is based on research with involuntary clients it gave me confidence that the approach I was taking with CN was appropriate.

Outcomes

Link worker accepted my assessment. It highlighted to me how thorough your assessment has to be to allow decisions to be justified.

Student evaluation of the use of this Critical Incident Analysis in supervision

My latest critical incident was with regard to work with a family where I had completed a Social Background Report [Report to the Reporter to the Children's Panel in Scotland]. The issue was non-attendance but there were lots of issues in the family, mum with mental health problems, etc. Although the report had been about non-attendance I wanted to do a more in-depth assessment and a care plan. My link worker had decided that our response should be a change of school placement. I felt that was inappropriate so I completed the critical incident analysis. It gave me the opportunity to reflect and to bring in theory, policy and process. I used it as a basis for supervision. My practice teacher agreed with my assessment, based on the critical incident analysis. He said it showed how I was using theory and not just personal opinion. It is good to write down these dilemmas and be forced almost to think through issues and not take things for granted.

Summary of student evaluations of the use of Critical Incident Analysis

All students were asked to evaluate how useful they had found using the Critical Incident Analysis in their practice learning. The key areas of usefulness were found to be that it: provided a structured approach to reflection and critical analysis; assisted the transfer of learning; helped the integration of theory and practice; helped the examination of practice issues; and was an aid to supervision.

Provides a structured approach to reflection and critical analysis

It clarified what it meant by reflection and analysis and helped me consolidate what I thought. It's logical and structured.

It assisted me to address things that I had missed and not analysed and taken as read. It helped me think while writing.

Assists transfer of learning

The focus on just one incident and going through the framework allows you to go into depth. You can use that technique in other aspects of your practice.

Getting feedback on the critical incident definitely helped me through the next situation, more as it was happening than after the event.

Helps the integration of theory and practice

It was the checking of what you were doing theoretically that was the main strength of the framework.

I decided in the end to go 'backwards' in that I started with a theory in the situation and then answered other aspects of the framework after that. I started with Trotter's [1999] pro-social modelling and role clarification and reflected on my practice.

Helps the examination of value issues

I had been told in my last placement that my reflection on value issues was not strong. The framework has definitely helped me here.

It was useful to address value issues. You could use the framework to explore and challenge and then it didn't appear too personal. It assisted me to develop my style as I can come over too dogmatic. It helps you consider what you think rather than what people want to hear.

Is an aid to supervision

My practice teacher had read it in advance ... It helped me get more out of the supervision session ... He had a structured response ... it was more formal ... you take it more seriously.

In the last supervision we chatted about it. It was a productive experience. Something that had come up. Particular themes that relate to my personality and how I deal with things. It is something that comes up repeatedly. I need to look at it in more detail. The procedure makes for a productive supervision and feedback. My style, my way of thinking is something that has been flagged up as areas to address.

In this chapter a Critical Incident Analysis Framework has been introduced and its potential uses described. The focus of this chapter has been on students' use of the framework. This framework given here was used with students in the final period of practice learning. If you are using the framework when starting practice learning, you might choose to focus on fewer aspects.

Exercise 1

If you are in a practice learning situation use the Critical Incident Analysis Framework explained in the chapter. You may choose to use it to assist your own critical analysis and integration of theory to practice or you may choose to share with a fellow student or your practice teacher.

If you are not in a practice learning situation at the moment, in order to prepare for the use of Critical Incident Analysis on practice learning, it is useful to practise its use with regard to a personal incident or with regard to learning in the academic setting. The framework below was devised for students on the first year of their social work course.

- Account of the incident:

    - What happened, where and when? Who was involved?

    - What was your role/involvement in the incident?

    - What was the context of this incident, i.e what led to the incident?

    - What was your intent and focus at this point?

- Initial responses to the incident:

    - What were your thoughts and feelings at the time of this incident?

    - What were the responses of other key individuals to this incident? If not known, what do you think these might have been?

- Issues and dilemmas highlighted by this incident:

    - Note any dilemmas related to this incident that you experienced.

    - Outline any values and/or ethical issues which are highlighted by this incident.

    - What took you by surprise or happened in a way you didn't expect?

- Outcomes:

    - What were the outcomes of this incident for the various participants?

    - Are there ways in which this incident has led (or might lead to) changes in how you think, feel or act in particular situations?

    - What are your thoughts and feelings now about this incident?

Exercise 2

One of the students in the research described how she used the Critical Incident Analysis with a service user. After the student had asked permission from the service user to use their interview for her Critical Incident Analysis the service user expressed interest and asked for a copy. On the student's next visit to the service user, the service user had completed her own Critical Incident Analysis which she said had helped her to think through the incident. This led the student to thinking that the Critical Incident Analysis could be more service user-friendly.

Construct a Critical Incident Analysis which you think would be user-friendly and explain your choice of questions.

Key learning points

- Critical Incident Analysis is a useful tool to analyse practice issues and dilemmas.

- It can be used as a focus for supervision.

- It is useful to assist the integration of theory and practice.

Further reading

Fook, J. (2002) *Social work: Critical theory and practice*, London: Sage.

Green Lister, P. and Crisp, B.R. (2007) 'Critical incident analysis: A practice learning tool for students and practitioners', *Practice* 19(1): 47–60.

11 Concluding remarks

The aim of this book is to provide students with a range of ways through which to develop their integration of theory and practice, critical reflection and understanding of the theories and processes which inform anti-oppressive practice. The tools and frameworks are presented for guidance and can be adapted according to the particular learning situation.

Critical reflection is a process which needs to be continually worked upon. Different academic and practice situations make particular demands on students, so the skills of transfer of learning are essential so that students can become fluent practitioners.

Chapters
5 & 6

Anti-oppressive practice is an equally important concept and process in social work education and practice. It has been shown in Chapters 5 and 6 that social work educators, practitioners and service users and carers have different views on what the key priorities should be. There is clearly no 'right way' to be anti-oppressive. Remaining questioning of given or dominant discourses, and critically reflecting on a situation from different perspectives, can assist students to do this, whilst at the same time they remain aware of the influences on their own value base.

Chapters
4 & 7

The integration of theory and practices encompasses both critical reflection and anti-oppressive approaches. It also requires students to 'get to grips' with theory. There is a plethora of social work texts and journals on assessment and intervention in social work. The research approach in Chapter 4 might assist students starting out in this area, and the process and framework for evaluating textbooks on assessment given in Chapter 7 may also be of use.

 In all, students have been introduced to three methods of intervention in Chapters 8 and 9, by demonstrating to student ways in they can begin to draw out key theoretical principles and critiques, and then engage in more in-depth critical analysis. Students' views on what assists in the integrating of theory and practice are the basis of Chapters 8 and 9, which drew heavily on the research that my colleagues and I have undertaken in social work education. Frameworks are offered which students have found to be helpful. As with all frameworks they may be adapted to suit each student's particular learning needs.

My acknowledgements again to all the students who participated in the various pieces of research which have informed this text.

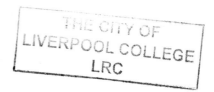

Bibliography

Adams, R. (2008) *Empowerment, participation and social work*, 4th edn, Basingstoke: Palgrave Macmillan.

Ahmad, B. (1990) *Black perspectives in social work*, London: Venture Press.

Bailey, R. and Brake, M. (1975) *Radical social work*, London: Edward Arnold.

Baldwin, N. and Walker, L. (2009) 'Assessment', in R. Adams, L. Dominelli and M. Payne (eds), *Social work: Themes, issues and critical debates*, 3rd edn, Basingstoke: Palgrave Macmillan.

Barn, R. (1993) *Black children in the public care system*, London: BT Batsford in association with BAAF.

Barnsdale, L. and Walker, M. (2007) *Examining the use and impact of family group conferencing*, Edinburgh: Scottish Executive.

Barron, J. (2009) *The survivor's handbook*, Women's Aid, via http://www.womensaid.org.uk/default.asp [accessed 27 August 2011].

Barry, M. (2007) *Effective approaches to risk management in social work: An international literature review*, Stirling: Scottish Government Publications.

Beresford, P. (2003) *It's our lives: A short theory of knowledge, distance and experience*, London: OSP for Citizen Press. Available online at: www.shapingourlives.org.uk/documents/ItsOurLives.pdf [accessed 27 August 2011].

Boud, D. and Feletti, G. (1997) *The challenge of problem-based learning*, 2nd edn, London: Kogan-Page.

Bowlby, J. (1963) 'Pathological mourning and child mourning', *Journal of the American Psychoanalytic Association*, 118: 500–41.

Bowlby, J. (1979) *The making and breaking of attachment bonds*, London: Tavistock.

Bowlby, J. (1982) *Attachment and loss*, London: Hogarth.

Bowlby, J. (1988) *A secure base: Clinical implications of attachment theory*, London: Routledge.

Braye, S. (2000) 'Participation and involvement in social care: An overview', in H. Kemshall and R. Littlechild (eds), *User involvement and participation in social care research informing practice*, London: Jessica Kingsley.

Bytheway, B. (1995) *Ageism*, Buckinghamshire: Open University Press.

Bywater, J. and Jones, R. (2007) *Sexuality and social work*, Exeter: Learning Matters.

Calder, M. (ed.) (2009) *Sexual abuse assessments: Using and developing frameworks for practice*, Lyme Regis: Russell Park.

Chand, A. (2000) 'The over-representation of black children in the child protection system: Consequences and solutions', *Child and Family Social Work*, 5(1): 67–86.

Chand, A. and Thoburn, J. (2006) 'Research review: Child protection referrals and minority ethnic children and families', *Child and Family Social Work*, 11(4): 368–77.

Charnley, H.M. and Langley, J. (2007) 'Developing cultural competence as a framework for anti-heterosexist practice: Reflections from the UK, *Journal of Social Work*, 7(3): 307–21.

Cherlin, A.J. (1997) 'A reply to Glenn: What's most important in a family textbook?', *Family Relations*, 46(3): 209–11.

Clark, A. (2007) 'Crisis intervention, in J. Lishman (ed.), *Handbook for practice learning in social work and social care*, 2nd edn, London: Jessica Kingsley.

Clifford, D. (1998) *Social assessment theory and practice: A multi-disciplinary framework*, Aldershot: Ashgate. Clifford, D. and Burke, B. (2009) *Anti-oppressive practice: Ethics and values in social work*, Basingstoke: Palgrave Macmillan.

Corcoran, J. and Pillai, V. (2009) 'A review of the research on solution-focused therapy', *British Journal of Social Work*, 39(2): 234–42.

Corrigan, P. and Leonard, P. (1978) *Social work practice under capitalism: A Marxist approach*, London: Macmillan.

Corden, J. and Preston-Shoot, M. (1987) 'Contract or Contrick? A reply to Rojek and Collins', *British Journal of Social Work*, 17(5): 535–43.

Corden, J. and Preston-Shoot, M. (1988) 'Contract or Contrick? A Postscript', *British Journal of Social Work*, 18(6): 623–34.

Cosis Brown, H. (1998) *Social work and sexuality: Working with lesbians and gay men*, Basingstoke: Macmillan.

Cosis Brown, H. and Cocker, C. (2011) *Social work with lesbians and gay men*, London: Sage.

Coulshed, V. and Orme, J. (2006) *Social work practice*, 4th edn, Basingstoke: Palgrave Macmillan.

Cowden, S. and Singh, G. (2007) 'The "user" friend foe or fetish: A critical exploration of user involvement in health and social care', *Critical Social Policy*, 27(1): 6–23.

Cree, V. (2000) 'The challenge of assessment', in C. Macaulay and V. Cree (eds), *Transfer of learning in professional and vocational education*, London: Routledge.

Crisp, B.R. and Green Lister, P. (2002) 'Assessment methods in social work education: Reviewing the literature', *Social Work Education* 21: 259–69.

Crisp, B.R., Anderson, M.R., Orme, J. and Green Lister, P. (2003) *Knowledge review: Learning and teaching in social work education*, London: Social Care Institute for Excellence.

Crisp, B.R., Anderson, M.R., Orme, J. and Green Lister, P. (2005) *Learning and teaching in social work education: Textbooks and frameworks on assessment*, London: Social Care Institute for Excellence.

Crisp, B.R., Anderson, M.R., Orme, J. and Green Lister, P. (2006) 'What we can learn about social work education from textbooks', *Journal of Social Work*, 6(3): 337–59.

Dalrymple, J. and Burke, B. (2006) *Anti-oppressive practice*, Maidenhead: McGraw-Hill.

Davies, H. and Kinloch, H. (2000) 'Critical Incident Analysis', in C. Macaulay and V. Cree (eds), *Transfer of learning in professional and vocational education*, London: Routledge.

de Shazer, S. (1985) *Keys to solutions in brief therapy*, New York: Norton.

de Shazer, S. (1988) *Clues: Investigating solutions in brief therapy*, New York: Norton.

de Shazer, S. (1991) *Putting difference to work*, New York: Norton.

de Shazer, S. (1994) *Words were originally magic*, New York: Norton.

Dermer, S.B., Hemesath, C.W. and Russell, C.S. (1998) 'A feminist critique of solution-focused therapy', *American Journal of Family Therapy* 26: 239–50.

Devore, W. and Schlesinger, E.G. (1991) *Ethnic-sensitive social work*, New York: Norton.

Doel, M. and Marsh, P. (1992) *Task-centred social work*, London: Ashgate.

Doel, M. and Shardlow, S.M. (2005) *Modern social work practice*, Aldershot: Ashgate.

Dominelli, L. (2002) *Feminist social work theory and practice*, Basingstoke: Palgrave.

Dominelli, L. (2008) *Anti-racist social work*, Basingstoke: Palgrave Macmillan.

Donnison, D. (2009) *Speaking to power: Advocacy for health and social care*, Bristol: Policy Press.

Dunn, R.S. (1996) *How to implement and supervise a learning style*, Alexandria, VA: Association for Supervision and Curriculum Development.

Entwistle, N. (1987) 'A model of the teaching–learning process', in J.T.E. Richardson, M.W. Eysenck and D.W. Piper (eds), *Student learning*, Milton Keynes: The Society for Research into Higher Education, Open University Press.

Entwistle, N. (1990) 'Teaching and the quality of learning in higher education', in N. Entwistle (ed.), *Handbook of educational ideas and practices*, London: Routledge.

European Brief Therapy Association (n.d.) 'SFBT evaluation list', http://www.ebta.nu/page2/page8/page8.html [accessed 15 September 2011].

Family Rights Group (n.d.) 'Family group conferences', http://www.frg.org.uk/fgc_model.html [accessed 26 August 2011].

Ferguson, I. and Lavalette, M. (2004) 'Beyond power discourse: Alienation and social work', *British Journal of Social Work*, 34(3): 297–312.

Fisher, A. and Scriven, M. (1997) *Critical thinking: Its definition and assessment*, Norwich: Centre for Research in Critical Thinking.

Fook, J. (2002) *Social work: Critical theory and practice*, London: Sage.

Freud, S. (1937) 'Construction of analysis', vol. 23 in J. Strachey (ed.), *The standard edition of the complete psychological works of Sigmund Freud*, London: Hogarth.

Gingerich, W.J. and Eisenhart, S. (2000) 'Solution-focused brief therapy: A review of outcome research', *Family Process* 3: 477–98.

Goldberg, E.M., Gibbons, J. and Sinclair, I. (1985) *Problems, tasks and outcomes: The evaluation of task-centred work in three settings*, London: Allen and Unwin.

Governance and Social Development Resource Centre (n.d.) 'Social exclusion', http://www.gsdrc.org/go/topic-guides/social-exclusion/social-exclusion-as-a-process [accessed 26 August 2011].

Graham, M. (2009) 'Reframing Black perspectives in social work: New directions', *Social Work Education*, 28(3): 268–80.

Green Lister, P. (2000) 'Mature students and transfer of learning', in C. Macaulay and V. Cree (eds), *Transfer of learning in professional and vocational education*, London: Routledge.

Green Lister, P. (2003) 'It's like you can't be a whole person, a mother who studies. Lifelong learning: Mature woman students with caring commitments', *Social Work Education* 2(2): 125–38.

Green Lister, P., Dutton, K. and Crisp, B.R. (2005) 'Assessment practices in social work education: A practice audit of Scottish universities providing qualifying courses', *Social Work Education*, 24(6): 693–711.

Green Lister, P. and Crisp, B.R. (2007) 'Critical Incident Analysis: A practice learning tool for students and practitioners', *Practice*, 19(1): 47–60.

Hall, G.S. (1904) *Adolescence: Its psychology and its relation to physiology, anthropology, sociology, sex, crime, religion and education*, vols 1 and 2, Englewood Cliffs, NJ: Prentice Hall.

Hafford-Letchfield, T. (2010) 'A glimpse of the truth: Evaluating "debate" and role play as a pedagogical tool for learning about sexuality issues on a law and ethic module', *Social Work Education* 29(3): 244–8.

Healy, K. (2005) *Social work theories in context: Creating frameworks for practice*, Basingstoke: Palgrave Macmillan.

Healy, K. and Mulholland, J. (2007) *Writing skills for social workers*, London: Sage.

Hepworth, D.H., Rooney, R.H. and Larsen, J.A. (2002) *Direct social work practice*, Pacific Grove, CA: Brooks Cole.

Heron, G. (2004) 'Evidencing anti-racism in student assignments: Where has all the racism gone?', *Qualitative Social Work*, 3(3): 277–95.

Hollis, F. (1964) *Social casework: A psychosocial theory*, New York: Random House.

Hollis, F. (1970) 'The psychosocial approach to the practice of casework', in R.W. Roberts and R.H. Nee (eds), *Theories of social casework*, Chicago: University of Chicago Press.

Hollis, F. and Woods, M.E. (1981) *Casework: A psychosocial approach*, 3rd edn, New York: Random House.

Honey, P. and Mumford, A. (1992) *The manual of learning styles*, Maidenhead: Peter Honey Publications.

Howe, D. (1995) *Attachment theory for social work practice*, Basingstoke: Macmillan.

Howe, D. (2000) 'Attachment', in J. Horwarth (ed.), *The child's world: Assessing children in need*, London: National Association for the Prevention of Cruelty to Children.

Hughes, B. (1995) *Older people and community care*, Buckinghamshire: Open University Press.

International Planned Parenthood Federation (2008) 'Sexual rights: An IPPF declaration', http://www.ippf.org/NR/rdonlyres/9E4D697C-1C7D-4EF6-AA2A-6D4D0A13A108/0/SexualRightsIPPFdeclaration.pdf [accessed 27 August 2011].

Jeyasingham, D. (2008) 'Knowledge/ignorance and the construction of sexuality in social work education', *Social Work Education*, 27(2): 136–51.

Jones, S. (2009) *Critical learning for social work students*, Exeter: Learning Matters.

Kemshall, H. (2002) *Risk, social policy and social work*, Buckinghamshire: Open University Press.

Kendrick, A. (2008) 'Black and minority ethnic children in residential child care', in A. Kendrick (ed.), *Residential child care: Prospects and challenges*, London: Jessica Kingsley.

Knowles, M.S. (1978) 'Innovations in teaching styles and approaches upon adult learning', *Journal of Education for Social Work*, 8: 32–9.

Kolb, D.A. (1976) *Learning styles inventory: Technical manual*, Newton, MA: Institute for Development Research.

Laming, H. (2003) *The Victoria Climbie inquiry CM 5730*, London: The Stationery Office.

Langan, M. and Lee, P. (1989) *Radical social work today*, London: Routledge.

Lee, J.A.B. (2001) *The empowerment approach to social work practice: Building the beloved community*, 2nd edn, New York: Columbia University Press.

Legault, G. (1996) 'Social work practice in situations of intercultural misunderstandings', *Journal of Multicultural Social Work*, 4: 49–66.

Macaulay, C. (2000) 'Transfer of learning', in C. Macaulay and V. Cree (eds), *Transfer of learning in professional and vocational education*, London: Routledge.

Mackay, R. (2007) 'Empowerment and advocacy', in J. Lishman (ed.), *Handbook for practice learning in social work and social care*, 2nd edn, London: Jessica Kingsley.

Marsh, P. and Doel, M. (2005) *The task-centred book*, London: Routledge.

Marshall, M., Philips, J. and Ray, M. (2005) *Social work with older people*, Basingstoke: Palgrave Macmillan.

Milner, J. (2008a) 'Working with people who are violent to their partners: A safety building approach', *Liverpool Law Review*, 29: 67–80.

Milner, J. (2008b) 'Domestic violence: Solution-focused practice with men and women who are violent', *Journal of Family Therapy*, 30: 29–53.

Milner, J. and O'Byrne, P. (2002) *Assessment in social work*, 2nd edn, Basingstoke: Palgrave Macmillan.

Milner, J. and O'Byrne, P. (2009) *Assessment in social work*, 3rd edn, Basingstoke: Palgrave Macmillan.

Minghella, E. and Benson, A. (1995) 'Developing reflective practice in mental health nursing through critical incident analysis', *Journal of Advanced Nursing*, 21: 205–13.

Monash University (n.d) 'Fieldwork documents', http://www.med.monash.edu.au/socialwork/fieldwork/fieldwork-placement-forms.html [accessed 27 August 2011].

Montalvo, F.F. (1999) 'The critical incident interview and ethnoracial identity', *Journal of Multicultural Social Work*, 7(3/4): 19–43.

Myers, J. (2007) *Theory into practice: Solution-focused approaches*, Lyme Regis: Russell House.

O'Connell, B. (2005) *Solution-focused therapy*, 2nd edn, London: Sage.

Oliver, M. (1990) *The politics of disablement*, 2nd edn, Basingstoke: Macmillan.

Oliver, M. and Sapey, B. (1999) *Social work with disabled people*, Basingstoke: Macmillan.

Orme, J. (2003) 'It's feminist because I say so!: Feminism, social work and critical practice in the UK', *Qualitative Social Work*, 2: 131.

Ornstein, A.C. (1994) 'The textbook-driven curriculum', *Peabody Journal of Education*, 3: 70–85.

Parad, H. (ed.) (1965) *Crisis intervention: Selected readings*, New York: Family Services Association.

Parker, J. and Bradley, G. (2003) *Social work practice assessment, planning and review*, Exeter: Learning Matters.

Parker, J. and Bradley, G. (2007) *Social work practice*, Exeter: Learning Matters.

Parton, N. (1998) 'Risk, advanced liberalism and child welfare: the need to discover uncertainty and ambiguity', *British Journal of Social Work*, 28 (1) 5–27.

Parton, N. and O' Byrne, P. (2000) *Constructive social work: Towards a new practice*, Basingstoke: Macmillan.

Payne, G. (2006) *Social divisions*, Basingstoke: Palgrave Macmillan.

Payne, M. (2005) *Modern social work theory*, 3rd edn, Basingstoke: Palgrave Macmillan.

Reid, W.J. (1978) *The task-centred system*, New York: Columbia University Press.

Reid, W.J. and Epstein, L. (1972) *Brief and extended casework*, New York: Columbia University Press.

Reid, W.J. and Hanrahan, P. (1981) 'The effectiveness of social work: Recent evidence', in E.M. Goldberg and N. Connolly (eds), *Evaluative research in social care*, London: Heinemann.

Reid, W.J. and Shyne, A. (1969) *Brief and extended casework*, New York: Columbia University Press.

Rich, A. and Parker, D. (1995) 'Reflection and critical incident analysis: Ethical and moral implications of their use within nursing and midwifery education', *Journal of Advanced Nursing*, 22: 1050–7.

Rojeck, C. and Collins, S. (1987) 'Contract or con trick?', *British Journal of Social Work*, 17(2): 199–211.

Rojeck, C. and Collins, S. (1988) 'Contract or con trick revisited: Comments on a reply by Corden and Preston-Shoot', *British Journal of Social Work*, 18(6): 611–22.

Sapey, B. (2009) 'Physical disability', in R. Adam, L. Dominelli and M. Payne (eds), *Critical practice in social work*, 2nd edn, Basingstoke: Palgrave Macmillan.

Schön, D.A. (1983) *The reflective practitioner: How professionals think in action*, London: Temple Smith.

Secker, J. (1993) *From theory to practice in social work*, Aldershot: Avebury.

Shaw, I., Briar-Lawson, K., Orme, J. and Ruckdeschel, R. (2010) *The Sage handbook of social work research*, London: Sage.

Sheldon, B. (2000) 'Cognitive behavioural methods in social care: A look at the evidence', in P. Stepney and D. Ford (eds), *Social work models, methods and theories*, Lyme Regis: Russell House.

Sigelman, C.K. and Rider, E.A. (2009) *Human development across the lifespan*, 6th edn, Belmont, CA: Wadsworth.

Smith, R. (2008) *Social work and power*, Basingstoke: Palgrave Macmillan.

Smale, G. and Tuson, G. with Biehal, N. and Marsh, P. (1993) *Empowerment, assessment, care management and the skilled worker*, London: National Institute for Social Work, HMSO.

Stainton, T. (2009) 'Learning disability', in R. Adam, L. Dominelli and M. Payne (eds), *Critical practice in social work*, 2nd edn, Basingstoke: Palgrave Macmillan.

Tanner, D. and Harris, J. (2008) *Working with older people*, London: Routledge.

Trevithick, P. (2005) *Social work skills: A practice handbook*, 2nd edn, Buckingham: Open University Press.

Tripp, D. (1993) *Critical incidents in teaching: Developing professional judgement*, London: Routledge.

Trotter, C. (1999) *Working with involuntary clients*, London: Sage.

Trotter, C. (2006) *Working with involuntary clients*, 2nd edn, London: Sage.

Trotter, J. and Gilchrist, J. (1996) 'Assessing DipSW students: Anti-discriminatory practice in relation to lesbian and gay issues', *Social Work Education*, 15(1): 75–82.

Walker, H. (2008) *Studying for your social work degree*, Exeter: Learning Matters.

Warren, J. (2007) *Service user and carer participation in social work*, Exeter: Learning Matters.

Index

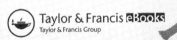